O, LET ME NOT GET ALZHEIMER'S, SWEET HEAVEN!

Why many people prefer death or active deliverance to living with dementia.

COLIN BREWER

SKYSCRAPER PUBLICATIONS

PREVIOUS BOOKS BY COLIN BREWER

Can social work survive
(with June Lait)

I'll see myself out, thank you
(with Michael Irwin)

Antabuse treatment for alcoholism
(with Emmanuel Streel)

O, let me not be mad, not mad, sweet heaven.
Keep me in temper: I would not be mad!

Shakespeare: King Lear.

LET ME NOT GET ALZHEIMER'S, SWEET HEAVEN!
Published by Skyscraper Publications Limited
20 Crab Tree Close, Bloxham, OX15 4SE
www.skyscraperpublications.com

First published 2019
Second printing 2019

Foreword copyright – Henry Marsh

Cover concept, design and typesetting
by chandlerbookdesign.com

Printed in the United Kingdom by CPI

ISBN-13: 978-1-911072-42-3

CONTENTS

Foreword by Henry Marsh   1

Preface   4

PART 1 THE PROBLEM: 9

1. Introduction   11

2. The Varieties and Trajectories of Dementia   27

3. Brain, Mind, Memory, Personhood and Identity in Dementia   38

4. What Dementia Looks Like   48

5. What Dementia Feels Like   64

6. Will You Still Need Me, Will You Tube-Feed Me, When I'm Ninety-Four?   72

7. What Do We Want? Euthanasia! When Do We Want It? As Soon As We Need 24-Hr Care!!   86

8. Even Worse Than Murder   114

9. Slippery Slopes: are they always a bad thing?   136

10. Leave it to Palliative Care and Hospices?   148

11. Families in Conflict   157

12. The Genetics Of Alzheimer's   166

13. Not Everyone Can be a Hero; Not Everyone Wants to be a Hero   172

14. The Really Difficult Future Debate   180

15. A Time to be Born and a Time to Die   189

PART 2 RESPONSES TO DEMENTIA: 197

16. Doing Nothing   199

17. Doing Something   204

18. Doing it Yourself   210

19. Doing it Abroad   221

20. A Final Word About Doctors and Our Privileged   234
Access to Self-Deliverance

APPENDIX 1   245

If Only Osvald Alving Could Have Had Penicillin

APPENDIX 2   249

Flow-chart for decision-making.

APPENDIX 3   251

Useful Addresses and Contacts

APPENDIX 4   254

Specimen advance decision/living will for dementia

APPENDIX 5   259

Blank Advance Decision/Living Will

Acknowledgements   263

About the Author   267

Index   269

Foreword by Henry Marsh

Evolution has equipped us with a profound fear of death – perhaps it is hard-wired into our brains. It may even be that this knowledge of our own mortality makes us unique among animals, though we can never know for certain what our fellow creatures think. Fear of death made evolutionary sense when our ancestors were at risk of dying when young, putting the survival of their children in jeopardy. Religious rituals and belief in an after-life are expressions of this deep fear. But how hard should we try to avoid death in old age, if we no longer believe in heaven or hell? Our fear of death becomes irrational – how can one be afraid of nothing? But fear of *dying* is a very different matter.

The scientific and industrial revolutions have brought great benefits to humankind, but also the double curse of climate change and long life. In a sense, both these problems are the two sides of the same coin – our insatiable desire to live. But we cannot live forever, however effective medicine becomes in the future. In the modern world, the two great diseases of old age are cancer and dementia. Treatment, even cure, of the first is often now possible, but despite intense research, no treatment has yet to be discovered for dementia, although perhaps one third of the risk is related to the way we live. Exercise, education and speaking more than one language, for instance, all have a protective effect, but increasing age remains the greatest risk. And nothing can stop us growing old.

Our ancestors all knew they would die, but only near the very end did they know *when* they would die. Modern, scientific medicine has made early diagnosis of both cancer and dementia possible. We may well now have a distressingly clear idea of what awaits us, even when we are still relatively well. Cancer brings the fear of pain and physical breakdown but dementia brings something much worse. Many of us will have had to witness a parent or elderly relative slowly sinking into the sad and vegetative state of the dement – a person we once loved who no longer has a mind or personality, and who has become an empty shell, a mere body. Few reasonable people, once diagnosed with dementia, can face this prospect with equanimity, whereas the quicker death sentence of terminal cancer, with good palliative care if you are lucky enough to get it, is perhaps less difficult to accept.

In several countries, Assisted Dying has become legal in recent decades. It comes in two forms, and varies from country to country. In its more limited form, doctors can help patients to die if they have a terminal prognosis of less than six months. In its less restricted form (as in the Netherlands, Belgium and Switzerland) it is also available for people who are faced by intractable suffering, such as dementia, provided that they still have the mental capacity to make an informed decision as to how they want their lives to end. As Colin Brewer explains in this powerful book, the case for Assisted Dying for those of us diagnosed with early dementia, is in many ways stronger than for those of us who will die within six months. Opinion polls in the UK have shown a large public majority in favour of legalizing Assisted Dying but a fierce minority (mainly of palliative care doctors and religious fundamentalists) remain implacably opposed to it. I will not recite here the arguments against their position but only observe that I find their attitude well-intentioned but profoundly paternalistic. The illegality of assisted dying in Britain is an undoubted cause of much suffering and its opponents have singularly failed to provide good evidence to justify this.

Read this book and ask yourself: what will you want for yourself, or for your family, if you are diagnosed with progressive, irreversible dementia? And what right have doctors, priests or politicians to order us how to live, or how to die?

Preface

My publisher's response after reading the first draft was: 'Could you possibly make the beginning a bit less bleak?' As will soon become clear if you haven't already come to that conclusion yourself, dementia – whether you're just thinking about it, are observing it in someone close to you, or have actually been diagnosed with it – is not something that's easy to be cheerful about but there is one dementia scenario that always brings out a smile. It's when I do a mental capacity assessment for someone with early dementia who plans to go to Dignitas or LifeCircle in Switzerland for an assisted suicide to ensure that their dementia never progresses beyond the early stage. The moment I confirm that they still have that precious capacity – simply put, that they understand what assisted suicide means, that they know they have dementia and understand what *that* means, that they have considered and rejected the alternatives and that their desire for assisted suicide is consistent – their pleasure and relief are immediate and obvious.

This is a book about one of the commonest and most serious dilemmas that many of us will face as we get older, unless we prefer not to think about it. If we survive until we are 85 – as most young and middle–aged people in Britain can now expect to do – nearly a third of us will be suffering from clinically obvious Alzheimer's or other varieties of dementia[1] The proportion increases remorselessly with each additional year, approaching 50% a decade later.[2] This is also a book about the most radical of the possible responses to that dilemma, which is to end our lives peacefully with suitable substances before the dementia becomes too severe and while we are still legally and physically able to do so. Attempting suicide has not been a crime in England for over half a century and the Church of England (though not of Rome) recently voted to abolish the indignities that were inflicted for over 1500 years on the bodies and souls of suicides and on the feelings of their grieving families. Suicide is one of the most distinctively and uniquely human of activities and usually one of the most shocking but given that we all have to die and that some dying scenarios are clearly much worse than others, in the case of dementia an increasing number of people are asking themselves whether it is better to die by deliberately ending our lives in a dignified, peaceful and painless way – with or without assistance – than by a progressive and unstoppable decline into dementia and the total destruction of our personalities and relationships that is dementia's end state. Sometimes, suicide is a very rational response to unrelievable medical conditions that do not just cause distress – to which the sufferer often adapts – but progressively remove from an individual life everything that the sufferer previously regarded as making it worth living, as dementia most certainly does.

---

[1] Skoog I, Nilsson L, Palmertz B, Andreasson LA, Svanborg A. A population-based study of dementia in 85-year-olds. N Engl J Med. 1993 Jan 21;328(3):153–8.

[2] Alexander M, Perera G, Ford L, et al. Age–Stratified Prevalence of Mild Cognitive Impairment and Dementia in European Populations: A Systematic Review. J Alzheimers Dis. 2015;48(2):355–9. doi: 10.3233/JAD–150168.

During the past decade, my retirement has been made even more interesting by doing a few psychiatric and mental capacity assessments for people who wanted to go to Dignitas or LifeCircle. Most of them suffered from forms of progressive paralysis such as motor neurone disease and a few had cancer – conditions that would not directly affect their brains or personalities as a rule but would be likely to end in increasingly unpleasant physical and mental pain and distress. Some hoped that their last weeks would not be as bad as they feared and just wanted the reassurance that if the best efforts of palliative care proved to be inadequate, there was an alternative. Just receiving that reassurance often visibly lifted their spirits. Others, especially the patients with motor neurone disease, knew that even the best palliative care could never relieve their fear of total paralysis, eventually affecting the muscles of breathing and causing gradual suffocation, and did not want to wait until the inevitable arrived.

A smaller but even more interesting group of potential travellers to Switzerland were not worried – at least not in the short or medium term – about the prospect of suffering severe pain or becoming totally paralysed and their illness was not at an advanced stage. What worried them was that they were in the early stages of Alzheimer dementia – an illness that would slowly and inexorably strip them not of the ability to move, hear or see but of even more important and fundamental abilities. All of them were or had been at least conventionally successful in their lives – sometimes more than that. Financially, they had been successful enough not to have much to worry about on that score either. Most were married and they had generally enjoyed good relationships with their spouses, siblings and children, most of whom seemed to have been equally fortunate in the lottery of life. All had either received a university education or had worked in jobs that required high levels of knowledge, experience and responsibility. If they were still working, they enjoyed their jobs. If they had retired, they seemed to be enjoying that too. They were resourceful, resilient and adaptable people and up to a point, I think they would have adapted to reduced mobility, hearing or vision at least as well as the average citizen; probably better.

Apart from the fact the fact that they were not doctors – a group whose rather special and possibly unfair advantages when faced with this dilemma are an important sub-theme of the book – they were people whose lives and antecedents had been very much like my own. They had either been fortunate or, if not, they had successfully overcome misfortune. Much of what they had achieved was a reflection of their intelligence, their formal or informal education, their choice of friends, partners and interests and of that crucial and almost defining ability of the educated, professional and managerial classes to defer gratification for long enough to acquire the means and position to enjoy it all the more. (And, some would add, the good fortune during their formative years to be exposed to peer–groups who shared and encouraged those aspirations.) What horrified them about Alzheimer's was the certainty of losing the ability to share, enjoy and discuss their ideas, experiences and affections. Often, they had campaigned for improvements in smaller or wider aspects of society and some were distinguished and honoured citizens. Life without travel or good food they could cope with. Life without books or music might be more problematic but life without conversation, argument, friendships or the sense of continuity and the recent memories necessary to sustain those things was not something they wanted to experience – or to inflict on others. They feared, and were right to fear, the loss of *themselves* – of their personalities, their identities and of their relationship with the world in which they had lived and adapted all their lives. They also feared the effect this progressive annihilation and loss would have on their nearest and dearest, with whom they would probably have no meaningful or enjoyable interaction for the last five years of their bodily life; sometimes longer. They wanted to go to Switzerland so that they could die in the presence of their family and friends when still recognizable as the person those onlookers had always known and loved. Their happiness when I was able to tell them that they still had the mental capacity that is a requirement of Swiss law was touching as well as obvious. When I subsequently contacted the families for a follow-up study, they almost always used words like 'beautiful' and 'uplifting' (as well as 'peaceful' and 'dignified') when describing their reactions to being present at the death. Even with hindsight, none of them thought that the alternative 'natural' death would have been better and none of them has needed any counselling or psychotherapy to come to terms with the experience.

PART 1

THE PROBLEM:

Alzheimer-type dementia slowly and inexorably destroys personalities, relationships, dignity and the ability to make decisions about how we live and how we die. It can also be miserable, terrifying and painful for sufferers and profoundly distressing for their families to watch.

1

Introduction

As life-expectancy steadily increases, most of us now worry more about getting dementia than about getting cancer.[3] That goes for doctors too. In the opening sentence of his universally praised and best–selling memoir *Admissions*, the neurosurgeon Henry Marsh writes: "…my most precious possession, which I prize above all my tools and books, and the pictures and antiques that I inherited from my family, is my suicide kit, which I keep hidden at home. It consists of a few drugs that I have managed to acquire over the years". And what's first on the list of his reasons for taking it out of its hiding place? "The early signs of dementia". In the same paragraph, he wonders if he would dare to use the drugs if it came to the crunch and notes that in countries where Voluntary Euthanasia or Medically Assisted Suicide are legal, many of the patients who are approved for the procedures do not activate them. That comment is statistically correct but it is (no doubt unintentionally) misleading, because it doesn't apply

---

[3] Batsch NL, Mittelman MS. 2012. World Alzheimer's Report 2012: Overcoming the stigma of dementia. Alzheimer's disease International: London, England. Available at: http://www.alz. co.uk/research/ WorldAlzheimerReport2012.pdf; (Accessed 28 Feb 2018.)

to dementia. It's true that the regular reports issued by Dignitas show that barely a fifth of British residents with terminal cancer who get the 'green light' actually go there in the end. Some die unexpectedly early of complications or sudden deterioration. A few get brain metastases that deprive them of mental capacity and some succeed in ending their lives without having to travel but many find that palliative care proves adequate and therefore don't need to go to the expense and the sometimes considerable trouble of getting themselves and their families to Switzerland. For those with early dementia, however, that is rarely true. I have assessed nearly every British dementia patient who applied to go to Switzerland in the last few years and only one of them had a change of mind, though two had left it too late and no longer had Mental Capacity by the time I saw them. I generally use capitals because it is a legal term with specific definitions in the Mental Capacity Act 2005 that include, in this context, the ability to understand information relevant to decisions about treatment, non-treatment or assistance to die and the reasonably foreseeable consequences of those decisions; "to retain that information; to use or weigh that information as part of the process of making the decision; and to communicate his decision (whether by talking, using sign language or any other means)". The Act adds that "The fact that a person is able to retain the information relevant to a decision for a short period only does not prevent him from being regarded as able to make the decision." Mental Capacity is also task specific, so that someone who lacks the Capacity to understand and make decisions about the complex financial details of a business that he or she owns may still have Capacity when it comes to simpler and much more easily understood decisions about treatment.

Henry Marsh's concern to avoid unpleasant ways of dying (which include losing his memory and identity to dementia) and his acquisition of the means to do so are common among doctors – certainly among his generation and mine – and it's clearly an old medical custom. The great 17th century physician William Harvey, the 'English Hippocrates' who discovered the circulation of the blood, had "a preparation of opium and I know not what, which he kept in his study to take, if occasion should serve, to put him out of his paine",[4] Not long ago, I had lunch with a well–known physician and his wife. I already knew from other people that he had recently been diagnosed with early Alzheimer's and he soon mentioned it, adding that he would end his life before the dementia progressed to the stage where he might no longer remain in control. It would be very easy, he added, to get the necessary medication by writing a prescription in his wife's professional name.[5] I shall return to this medical privilege at the end of the book.

In 2016, dementia – mostly of the Alzheimer type – became the commonest cause of death in England and Wales. Although many people think of dementia as a brain disorder, it makes its presence known by its disturbing effects on thinking and behaviour and therefore it comes into the category of what most people call 'mental' or 'psychiatric' illness (or more euphemistically, 'mental health conditions'). There will be more on the brain–mind question in Ch 3. People with mental illness are sometimes said to have 'lost their mind'. That loss can be temporary (as with an acute psychosis) or permanent (as with severe chronic schizophrenia); and also as with most types of dementia. It is by far the most untreatable as well as now one of the commonest forms of adult mental illness.

It's not easy to be positive about dementia. Bipolar patients on a moderate high are often entertaining and creative and much good poetry and literature (though a smaller amount of good

---

[4] Keynes G. The life of William Harvey. 1966. Oxford OUP. p. 436.

[5] In the event, he had a fatal heart attack before his dementia reached that stage. Unlike most heart attacks, it was regarded by his family as a blessing, on balance.

music) has been written in the manic phase of manic–depressive illness. When manic patients are so happy, it almost seems a pity when a psychiatrist has to be called in because they're making everyone else miserable. Writers emerging from severe depression sometimes distil masterpieces from their voyages to the abyss. A decade before she drowned herself, the manic–depressive Virginia Woolf wrote to her friend the composer Dame Ethel Smythe: "As an experience, madness is terrific I can assure you, and not to be sniffed at; and in its lava I still find most of the things I write about. It shoots out of one, everything shaped, final, not in mere driblets as sanity does". Schizophrenics can have interesting and grandiose delusions (or paint fantastical cats, like Louis Wain) and the products of Vincent van Gogh's descent into what was probably absinthe–fuelled insanity continue to amaze us. Entire religions have been founded and written about by people whose proclaimed messages from God were really the result of epileptic electrical storms in their temporal lobes. In depressing contrast, there's really not much to be said for dementia. It is written about – and occasionally painted – by the non–demented but eventually it doesn't *produce* any art. There's no such thing as 'Alzheimer Lit', at least not if by that term we mean things written or composed by people with well–established Alzheimer's Disease – or any of the other varieties of dementia, of which Alzheimer's is actually not the worst. Books are written and paintings executed by people in the early-to-moderate stages of the disease but nobody fights bravely through Alzheimer's to the other side against all odds and then writes about the experience. There *is* no other side.

One of those varieties of dementia, now extremely rare in developed countries thanks to penicillin, is General Paresis of the Insane (GPI) – tertiary syphilis affecting the brain.[6]

---

[6] 'Paresis' means weakness. GPI can cause general weakness but not general paralysis.

It used to be as common as Alzheimer's is now and was probably what caused Robert Schumann to spend his last two years in an asylum.[7] During that time, the normally productive composer managed only a few short and pathetic pieces that are of pathological rather than musical interest. GPI caused art–dealer Theo van Gogh to follow his brother Vincent into an asylum and then death six months later. The fictional Osvald Alving in Ibsen's play 'Ghosts' realises that he is losing his mind because of GPI and makes it clear to his horrified mother that he plans to commit suicide with morphine, precisely because he cannot trust her to do the job for him when he can no longer do it for himself. "But this is so horribly revolting", says Osvald. "To be turned into a helpless child again. To have to be fed, to have to be ... Oh! It doesn't bear talking about."That prospect presumably explains why half the respondents in a survey of family caregivers of people with dementia in Québec "believed that the fear of living the advanced stages of Alzheimer disease should be considered as unbearable suffering".[8]

A steadily increasing number of people seem to be having – and voicing – the same thoughts as the Québec caregivers and young Osvald, though Ibsen's play ends with that particular question still unresolved. Some of them go to Switzerland for assisted suicide while they still retain the capacity to choose both the way they will die and the quality of the last months or years of their lives. We shall meet some of them later. Others don't need to travel because they live in countries where

---

[7] What's a vigorous young Bohemian to do with his libido when the father of his 15-year-old girl-friend understandably forbids all contact until she reaches 21? Syphilis did for Schubert, too

[8] Bravo G, Rodrigue C, Arcand M. et al Are Informal Caregivers of Persons With Dementia Open to Extending Medical Aid in Dying to Incompetent Patients? Findings From a Survey Conducted in Quebec, Canada. Alzheimer Dis Assoc Disord. 2017 Dec 27. doi: 10.1097/WAD.0000000000000238

assisted suicide or voluntary euthanasia are legal options in early dementia; or because they find out from the internet how to end their lives without assistance; or – like Henry Marsh – already possess the means and the know-how. As well as being 'turned into, a helpless child again', dementia often means frightening hallucinations and delusions before the more purely vegetative phase sets in but whereas people usually died within a year or two of the onset of GPI, the average diagnosis-to-death interval for Alzheimer's is just over seven years, of which nearly half is likely to be in the moderate-to-severe stage. That means a serious, progressive and eventually total failure to initiate or maintain ordinary human relationships with other people. For some types of dementia, the period is even longer. There's no penicillin for Alzheimer's and no sign of one any time soon. As I write this early in 2018, a major British pharmaceutical company has just announced that it is withdrawing from Alzheimer research. It's an optimist's nightmare on which Dr Pangloss himself would have found it hard to put a positive spin. Even – for when Alzheimer comes, things can only get worse – with help from Tony Blair.[9]

Yet if you take a look at the websites of the Alzheimer Society UK and its equivalents in other countries, they are full of smiling faces. Obviously, such organisations want to provide hope and comfort as well as information and smiles are not hard to come by in the early stages, though many early-stage patients show confusion and distress and some experience frightening mood changes or delusions. However, the absence of images showing the typical manifestations of middle-stage and advanced dementia is both telling and misleading. Where are the patients sitting blank and indifferent to the efforts of staff to engage them, or – in the final stages – bedridden, skeletal

---

[9] New Labour's theme song in the 1997 election that first made Mr Blair prime minister was 'Things can only get better'.

and looking very much like the survivors and corpses found by the liberators of Belsen? Where, too, are the patients' distraught, despairing and sleepless spouses and children? In a later chapter, I note a comment by the carer of someone affected by a different type of chronic disability, who told researchers that it is "taboo" in that particular community "to say anything negative" about life with an affected family member. Something similar seems to influence Alzheimer activists. Patients and their families need to be prepared for worst-case scenarios as well as best-case ones. In reality, when Alzheimer patients eventually die, it is nearly always seen as a merciful release for everyone. However much Alzheimer victims may have been genuinely loved before both their brains and their personalities withered away, professions of love and affection sound ever more hollow when spouses, children, grandchildren and old friends are met in the last two or three years of the disease with a blank and blandly smiling face at best. At worst, they are met with screams of anger, terror or pain; or a confused muttering and picking at the bedclothes; or complete silence and closed eyes as food is squirted from a large syringe into a Percutaneous Endoscopic Gastrostomy or PEG – a sort of mini-colostomy in reverse that allows food to go straight into the stomach without needing to be chewed, or swallowed; or tasted; or enjoyed.

Shortly after I started writing this book, a British judge ruled that a woman with a particularly unpleasant type of dementia due to Huntington's Disease could be allowed to die by not putting any food or water into the PEG that had been keeping her body alive for over a year He added that in future, it would not be necessary for the doctors in charge of similar patients to seek a court ruling, provided that both the doctors and the patient's family agreed that feeding should cease.[10]

---

[10] www.theguardian.com/lifeandstyle/2017/sep/20/right-to-die-court-decision-severe-illnesses-life-support

In July 2018, Britain's Supreme Court ruled that this applied to patients in a Persistent Vegetative State as well. It can take a week or so for people to die from dehydration, though perhaps only a few days if other vital organs are also failing but it is not a nice death for families (or doctors and nurses) to witness, unless the patient is generously sedated.

Numerous surveys – discussed in Chapter 7 – confirm that many people don't want to spend years in a state of progressive physical, intellectual and personality disintegration before death delivers them and their families from one of the commonest, most prolonged and most distressing ordeals that modern life can throw at us. If they do become severely demented and even if their dementia is far from terminal, a large majority would refuse any treatment that prolongs their lives. If they were to get pneumonia or a heart attack, most hope that it would prove fatal and a majority in Britain would be grateful if their doctors speeded things up. This book is aimed partly at those many people and families but also at the many doctors and nurses who – often against their compassionate instincts – are too fearful of becoming embroiled in exhausting legal or professional proceedings (or twitter-storms) to question the system, except in private conversation or contemplation. The fact that doctors quite often use their special knowledge and access to appropriate medicines to escape these indignities themselves is an additional argument that their patients should be similarly empowered.

I hope this book will stimulate debate about the alternatives to waiting for dementia to take its 'natural' course. The quotation marks are there because what used to be the 'natural' course is often prolonged by months or years when acute infections or heart problems that might have cut it short not so long ago are now successfully treated. That happens very often, even when dementia is not merely advanced but truly terminal and when patients had clearly and consistently indicated that they wouldn't want any treatment other than pain relief and sedation. This will be a recurrent theme and it gets a separate discussion in Ch 7. In early dementia, the alternatives boil down to Voluntary Euthanasia (VE), and its very close relation Medically-Assisted Rational Suicide (MARS) or Unassisted Rational Suicide (URS). The 'rational' prefix serves to remind us that what one might call 'ordinary' suicide (both intended and completed) is almost invariably driven by failures or losses, and is often youthful, impulsive and poorly thought out. It is heavily over–represented at the bottom of the social, educational and employment pyramid, as is the alcoholism or other drug abuse (and personality disorder) that often fuels it. As the most thorough examination of the reasons for a whole century's worth of suicide has shown, the large majority of successful suicides are due to understandable unhappiness – understandable in terms of an individual's development, personality, habits, relationships, environment, hopes, expectations and to sheer bad luck (or whatever other name we choose to give to the reverse of serendipity).[11] 'Mental illness' accounts for no more than 20–30%, unless we define it so broadly – as some psychiatrists, journalists and patients evidently do – that it includes the unhappiness of bereavement, divorce and other misfortunes. Some of that 20–30% has demonstrated its persistent failure to respond to psychiatric treatment over many unhappy years.

This type of exit from life could hardly be more different from the desire for death that is typical of older people who have usually led reasonably happy and successful lives – both economically and emotionally – but are now facing conditions,

---

[11] Weaver J. Sorrows of a century: interpreting suicide in New Zealand 1900–2000. Montreal, McGill–Queens, 2014. Weaver's team examined every document submitted to New Zealand coroners for the inquests of all suicides in the even years of the entire 20th century. Their conclusions are almost certainly valid for British society, which has many similarities and has experienced similar recent changes.

including dementia, for which no acceptable treatment or palliation exists. Since these differences are absolutely crucial to any debate, I have tabulated them below.

Table 1: Bad/ordinary versus Good/rational/suicide

	Bad/Ordinary/Unassisted	Good/Rational/Assisted/VE
Age	15 upwards	Mostly over-65
If they had lived	Many would survive for many years of reasonably happy life	Most would survive only for weeks or months* – sometimes years – of increasing misery.
Family response	Usually very distressed and wanted them to live. Often isolated.	Often happy that they had had a good death and didn't want alternative. Rarely isolated
Mental state	Always unhappy and often pathological	Usually happy and rational
Psychiatric diagnosis	Common/relevant	Unusual/irrelevant
Die alone?	Nearly always	Usually die in company
Past history	Often much unhappiness and failure	Usually prosperous, happy and successful lives
Motive or major factor	Often shame, crime, debt, failure, relationships, isolation	Never shame, crime, or relationships, and very rarely isolation.
Impulsive?	Often	Never
Intoxicated before attempt?	Often	Never

★ Obviously, 'weeks or months' applies mainly to conditions like cancer and motor neurone disease but there is often a similar period from the diagnosis of early dementia to loss of Mental Capacity and thus the possibility of VE where permitted, or of MARS in Switzerland.

A recent position statement by the American Association of Suicidology[12] includes most of the comparisons in my list but adds that "Ending one's life with the assistance of a physician and with the understanding of one's family is often viewed more as 'self-preservation' than 'self-destruction', acting to die while one still retains a sense of self and personal dignity, before sedation for pain or the disease itself takes away the possibility of meaningful interaction with those around one".

Rather than frequently repeating various acronyms, I generally use the term 'deliverance' to refer to those alternatives. That includes self-deliverance – Unassisted Rational Suicide (URS) – unless it needs emphasizing specifically. 'Deliverance'[13] is a fine old word and one of its oldest meanings refers to avoidance (as in 'deliver us from evil'). While 'evil' can mean both doing and experiencing bad things, dementia is undoubtedly a great evil. Another term I use to cover the methods that involve doctors at some level is Medical Assistance in Dying, which is its official title in recent Canadian legislation. It makes a neat acronym – MAID – but unlike 'deliverance', it cannot include the Do-it-Yourself variety. As Michael Irwin and I have argued elsewhere,[14] the differences between the three types of deliverance are differences of style rather than substance. In essence, they resemble decisions about how to redecorate a room in your home: you can do it yourself (as many people do) but it often saves trouble, anxiety and messy mistakes to get the job done by a professional decorator, especially if you are not as agile as you used to be.

---

[12] Statement of The American Association of Suicidology: "Suicide" is not the same as "Physician Aid In Dying" Approved October 30, 2017

[13] 'the action of being rescued or set free' (OED). First recorded use in the 14th C.

[14] Brewer C, Irwin M. (Eds) I'll See Myself Out, Thank You. The arguments for rational suicide. Newbold on Stour, Warwickshire. Skyscraper. 2015. 131–4

For reasons that probably reflect the unusually prominent place of religion in the USA's public discourse, professional assistance in deliverance – in the small but increasing number of states in the USA where it is currently legal – has taken the form of supplying rather than administering lethal drugs: i.e. Medically Assisted Rational Suicide rather than Voluntary Euthanasia. In that scenario, the professional will, as it were, supply the pharmacological equivalent of some rather basic paint or wallpaper and will tell you how to apply it but will not assist your efforts or advise you about the more sophisticated techniques that he knows about (and would probably use himself if he had to). For the real Do-It-Yourself version (Unassisted Rational Suicide), you will have to get all the information and materials from reading about it, from friends, or from personally reinventing this particular wheel unaided.

In Western Europe, Colombia[15] and countries in the non–US, 'Old Commonwealth' Anglosphere that allow medical assistance (or aid) in dying, the preference among patients is usually for doctors to administer the drugs rather than just supplying or prescribing them. We should not forget that the first legislature that allowed Voluntary Euthanasia *de jure* as well as *de facto* (as it had been in the Netherlands since the 1980s) was the Parliament of Australia's Northern Territory in 1996. Several patients – including a nurse – travelled there from other parts of Australia before opponents in the Federal Parliament used their power to overturn the law because the Territory's legal status was slightly different from that of other Australian states. Generally this Western European-Old Commonwealth Anglosphere model that allows or requires Voluntary Euthanasia, means that the doctor can do the whole

---

[15] Historically and culturally, Colombia is probably closer to Spain than to the USA and its law requires medication to be administered by a doctor, not the patient.

job for you and also, like the decorator, offers a wider range of techniques, because the lethal drugs can be given by intravenous or subcutaneous injection, which is quicker, more pleasant and about as foolproof as anything human can be. It removes any fear (however misplaced) that self–administered medication may be vomited, or not work. In their truly final moments, surely people should not have to worry about that, or struggle to ingest medication if they are very weak or have difficulty swallowing, which often happens in advanced neurological conditions like motor neurone disease. Another advantage of Voluntary Euthanasia is that breathing is usually stopped within a minute of unconsciousness occurring by the injection of a separate drug. Death – permanent cardiac arrest – can then be confirmed a few minutes later. With self–administered oral medication, breathing may continue intermittently but noisily for many minutes and occasionally hours after swallowing barbiturates (the usual lethal drug) and death is correspondingly delayed. That can be very distressing for those gathered around the death-bed, who may not understand that the patient is deeply unconscious and beyond discomfort.[16] At one Swiss organization – LifeCircle – the medication is always administered intravenously but while a doctor inserts the needle into a vein, it is the patient who initiates the infusion by opening a small valve that starts the flow. It is a modern version of that famous mediaeval needle on whose point the number of angels that could theoretically dance was hotly disputed. The dedicated

---

[16] In Winchester in 1993, a terminally ill patient of Dr Nigel Cox refused further treatment and was given – probably quite legally under the 'double effect' principle and with the full agreement of the patient and her watching family members – what amounted to terminal sedation. Although she was unconscious, her noisy terminal breaths were distressing the family and Dr Cox therefore administered a drug to stop her heart. That led to his prosecution and conviction for attempted murder – for which he was not imprisoned and only briefly suspended from work.

doctor who founded the organization, and still practices mainly in palliative care, regards the question of who opens the valve as extremely important. Much as I respect her, I doubt whether most of her patients take the same view, especially if they find valves difficult to open. When patients can choose between self-administered or doctor-administered medication, as in most of Canada, Belgium and The Netherlands, nearly all of them (99.9% in Canada[17]) seem to prefer a doctor to have ultimate control of the procedure. Similar German and Swiss laws on assisted suicide have existed for a century but whereas Swiss doctors are allowed to prescribe barbiturate sedatives in lethal doses, it is currently difficult for German doctors to do so, or for German pharmacists to dispense them. In response, German right-do-die societies have developed alternative methods, using drugs that are more easily obtainable including one that does not need a prescription in many countries. Death is not so rapid as with pentobarbitone but seems to be peaceful and certain.[18]

When it comes to conditions like cancer and motor neurone disease, the arguments for making deliverance legal are both familiar and widely supported by very large majorities of citizens in most developed countries – now over 90% in the most recent British opinion survey[19]. In both of those conditions, patients generally retain their mental capacity, in both the legal and everyday meanings of the term. If they

---

[17] Downey J. Recent developments and the future of MAID in Canada. Paper presented at the 3rd International conference on end of life law, ethics, policy and practice. Ghent. March 7th – 9th 2019.

[18] I have heard from more than one Swiss informant that the assisted suicide law had military origins and allowed fellow-officers to give a revolver (and presumably the traditional bottle of whisky) to an officer who had disgraced his regiment without their being penalized. I have not seen documentary evidence for this claim and different sources date the law's enactment to the 1890s, 1918 or 1942.

[19] https://www.theguardian.com/society/2019/mar/03/legalise-assisted-dying-for-terminally-ill-say-90-per-cent-of-people-in-uk

wish to hasten their deaths, they can at least refuse treatment, food or fluids or consider the Swiss option (if they can afford it) but one of the defining features of advanced dementia is that it destroys mental capacity. In the case of Alzheimer's, the destruction usually happens at least four or five years before death. That makes dementia a special case because it means that if the natural course of the disease is to be interrupted by deliverance or self-deliverance (or conscious refusal of food and water for the very stoic or very desperate) it must usually be interrupted not when the distressing symptoms reach a personal peak of severity and intolerability but before they get to that point. In the Benelux countries, Voluntary Euthanasia in early dementia is acceptable but in some cases, it has been extended to patients who have lost mental capacity, provided that they had previously made a very clear written request for VE to be carried out when Capacity had been lost or when dementia was advanced but not yet terminal. As we shall see, that is an arrangement that many British citizens would welcome. There is also considerable support for it in several other countries where surveys have been done and the supporters include physicians, nurses and carers as well as potential patients. However, when even restricted, US-style legislative proposals have repeatedly failed by large majorities to be enacted in Westminster, not to mention the current political uncertainties, it might prove optimistic to expect any British deliverance laws at all within the next ten years. On the other hand, that means there will be plenty of time for the public debate to which I hope this book will usefully contribute.

Dementia is also special because, probably more than any other common adult condition, it causes great unhappiness (and stress) to family and friends over a period of many years because the personality – and thus the possibility of communicating and exchanging affection, experiences and ideas – dies long before the body does. The unhappiness is not reduced and may even be increased when patients are no longer able to appreciate the distress that their condition is causing to others, or to remember the distress they themselves may have experienced a day ago; or an hour ago; or five minutes ago. Finally, dementia is 'special' because while it is now the commonest cause of death in most regions of the United Kingdom, if we include patients with dementia whose deaths were recorded as primarily due to some other illness such as pneumonia, dementia is probably an important factor in as many as a quarter of all UK deaths. It is the elephant in the room and a very large (and growing) elephant at that. My aim is to describe the elephant, tame it and – perhaps – make it grow more slowly.

2

The Varieties and Trajectories of Dementia

Alzheimer's is not the worst.

The usual progress of Alzheimer's disease – and of most other dementias – is a slow and steady decline into memory loss, fatuity, personality change or disintegration, misidentification, confusion, social withdrawal, weakness, immobility, incontinence and silence. Quite often, mood changes, aggression or psychotic symptoms, such as delusions and hallucinations, are added to the mix. As with all illnesses, some patients have a more (or less) rapid course than the majority but in a recent British post–mortem study, the average duration of the disease after diagnosis was 7.1 years. 25% of cases died within four years, 50% within seven years, and 75% within ten (which means that 25% of cases lasted more than ten years from onset to death).[20] Current drugs for Alzheimer's can make that decline even slower and few patients would not want to give them a trial but they can only delay the inevitable. They cannot prevent it. Developments in genetic testing may make it

---

[20] Armstrong RA. Factors determining disease duration in Alzheimer's disease: a post-mortem study of 103 cases using the Kaplan–Meier estimator and Cox regression. . 2014;2014:623487.

easier to predict both the likelihood of developing Alzheimer's and the speed of decline, though if Huntington's Disease (see below) is any guide, many actual or potential sufferers will not wish to know either of those predictions.

There are two main types of dementia and both are common. The first *degenerative* type involves a general and progressive shrinkage (or *atrophy*) of the largest part of the brain – the cerebral hemispheres. The hemispheres contain the most important brain areas for speech, language, vision, hearing, voluntary movement, and memory.

The frontal part of the cerebral hemispheres – the frontal lobes situated immediately behind the forehead – is proportionately larger in humans than in any other animal and is almost certainly what makes us distinctively human. The frontal lobes are crucial for what are often called 'higher functions' – things like judgment, planning, self-awareness, empathy with other creatures, the more subtle social skills, awareness of mortality and the ability to philosophise. In dementia, these higher functions gradually disappear, as does memory. (So, intriguingly, does the ability to respond to placebo effects.) Both sides of the brain are equally affected in degenerative dementias and the atrophy is therefore symmetrical. Alzheimer's is the classic example, accounting for around 75% of dementias. In fronto-temporal dementia, the frontal and temporal lobes are affected sooner than other brain areas but the end result is identical. Degeneration makes the grooves (or *sulci*) on the surface of the hemispheres become larger as the brain shrinks and the outer layer of grey matter – the *cortex*, containing many of the heads (or *nuclei*) of the brain cells – becomes smaller in volume. Most cells in the body are microscopic in size and round or cylindrical in shape but many brain cells have long tails (or *axons*) that can extend from the *nuclei* in the brain right down to the lower portion of the spinal cord.

NORMAL AND ALZHEIMER'S BRAINS COMPARED

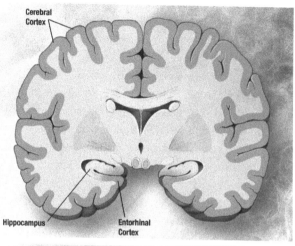

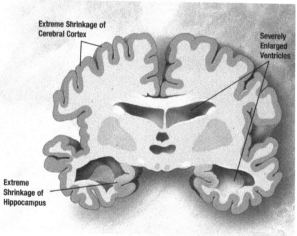

Figure 1

The normal brain, at the top, has small ventricles (internal cavities) and the sulci (grooves) in the cortex are narrow. In the shrunken brain of someone with advanced Alzheimer dementia, lower image, the sulci become wider and the ventricles are enlarged. The space left by the shrinkage fills with cerebro-spinal fluid.

The underlying white matter of the brain, which is mainly composed of axons (also called 'nerve fibres' in everyday speech) and represents most of the volume of the hemispheres, also atrophies.   At a post–mortem examination, white matter atrophy in the intact brain is not so obvious to the naked eye but its shrinkage means that the cavities inside the brain (the *ventricles*) become larger. The extra space in both the enlarged sulci and the enlarged ventricles simply fills up with the cerebro–spinal fluid (CSF) that surrounds the brain and spinal cord and both the atrophy and the enlarged ventricles can be seen and measured on CT or MRI scans. The rate at which Alzheimer and other degenerative dementias progress varies from one patient to another but is usually fairly steady for an individual patient, with no sudden changes from one day or one week to the next.

The second type of dementia typically involves increasingly numerous areas of focal, localised damage (or *lesions*) in small and separate areas of the brain in both the cortex and the white matter. The usual cause is a blockage of the small arteries that supply these areas by a blood–clot (or *thrombus*) or 'hardening of the arteries' (*atheroma*), causing the death or *infarction* of that particular area of the brain. How blood is distributed within the brain differs from the way it is distributed within most other organs. For example, if a small artery supplying part of a muscle gets blocked, blood can often flow from another small artery nearby to make up for it but that doesn't happen in the brain, or the heart. There is no communication between the small 'end arteries' of one area and the adjacent area.

Sometimes, the lesions are caused not by blockage but by localized bleeding or *haemorrhage* from a break in the wall of a small artery. Either way, these mini–haemorrhages and mini–infarcts can be thought of as mini-strokes. The brain can often adapt to a few small lesions but as the number and/or size of the lesions increases, the effect eventually resembles the generalized damage of Alzheimer dementia. This variety is usually called vascular or arteriosclerotic dementia. It accounts for 15-20% of dementias and it differs in some important ways from the Alzheimer types. The first is that brain function in vascular dementia can get much worse quite suddenly if the next stroke is not a mini-stroke but something bigger that takes out a significant amount of brain tissue, or affects an area that is particularly important.

The second is that these small and not-so-small strokes often affect brain areas that deal with movement and speech, which may be significantly impaired before a more general loss of intellect, higher functions and memory are obvious. There may also be partial recovery from a larger stroke as some brain cells that are damaged but not dead resume their functions. From the point of view of those who want deliverance before dementia removes their Mental Capacity, it is more difficult to plan for vascular dementia than for the Alzheimer type, because the course is less predictable, though it tends to be shorter.

Finally, while – in the present state of knowledge – there is not much that can be done to prevent Alzheimer's and similar dementias, vascular dementia is often associated with high blood pressure and the clogging of arteries with atheroma. The early detection and treatment of hypertension (high blood pressure), together with statins and anti–clotting drugs such as aspirin, may delay or avoid both the onset and the progress of vascular dementia, though anti–clotting drugs carry some risk of strokes from bleeding into the brain rather than from blockage of brain arteries.[21] Unfortunately, there is no law of

---

[21] There is a relatively high incidence of vascular dementia in Trinidad (Davis G, Baboolal N, Mc Rae A, Stewart R. Dementia prevalence in a population at high vascular risk: the Trinidad national survey of ageing and cognition. BMJ Open. 2018 Feb 22;8(2):e018288. doi: 10.1136/bmjopen–2017–018288). This may reflect the high prevalence of diabetes, among other factors.

God or Nature that prevents people from having both main types of dementia simultaneously and both of them become commoner with increasing age.

The remaining 5-10% of dementias is a mixed bag of degenerative brain diseases like Huntington's Disease, fronto-temporal dementia (sometimes called Pick's disease) and Lewy body dementia. I won't go into them in any detail but they all end in the same way. Here are some brief summaries. In Pick's disease, personality change, mood disturbances or even psychotic symptoms like paranoid delusions and hallucinations, often occur before any form of memory loss, unlike Alzheimer's, where memory loss is usually the first sign. Second only to Alzheimer's in prevalence, Pick's disease accounts for 20% of young-onset dementia cases. Lewy body dementia is the fourth commonest variety after Alzheimer's and vascular. It tends to start younger but the average diagnosis-to-death interval is about the same as with Alzheimer's. Corticobasal Degeneration (CBD) or Corticobasal Ganglionic Degeneration is one of the rarer degenerative dementias. CBD symptoms typically begin between 50-70 years of age, and the average disease duration is six years. It is characterized by marked disturbances in both movement and cognitive function. In Progressive Supranuclear Palsy, speech and visual impairments often appear relatively early in the course of the disease.

Research increasingly indicates that repeated head trauma can either initiate an Alzheimer–type dementia or cause a separate dementing process. It used to be thought that only professional boxers developed what was called *dementia pugilistica*, but it can affect amateurs as well and repeated heading in football has also been implicated. Regular heavy alcohol consumption or even a single prolonged binge can cause irreversible brain damage, sometimes as early as the 20s and 30s. Korsakov syndrome – the most dramatic variety because of its sudden onset – does not usually progress if drinking stops but heavy drinking may also exacerbate or initiate an Alzheimer–type dementia.

As well as the cerebral hemispheres, some of these rarer dementias also involve the *basal ganglia* in the mid–brain and the cerebellum. Those parts are important for controlling movement and tremor is often a prominent additional feature. Dementia is not a routine feature of Parkinson's disease but may be a late manifestation in a significant proportion of patients and is found in about half the cases that start after the age of 80.[22] Following the 'mad cow disease' crisis of the 1990s, the widely-predicted epidemic of new-variant Creutzfeld-Jakob disease in British beef-eaters was either a false alarm or will not show itself for another decade or two because of the very long incubation period for this virus-like prion brain infection that caused dementia in several British teenagers. (Prion brain disease was first recorded in the remote Fore tribe in New Guinea, who ritually consumed the brains of their dead.) Almost all of these dementias are progressive – some more rapidly than others – and currently have no cure. There have been some promising results of gene-modification in one type of rare and inheritable dementia but even if it proves a real advance (which will need several years of study to confirm and evaluate) it seems unlikely to be of use in other types. Unless interrupted by other lethal illnesses, or by deliverance, they all end in the situation that so horrified Osvald Alving and clearly horrifies many of today's citizens as well.

Alzheimer's is bad enough but it is not the worst of the dementias – a distinction which probably belongs to that uniquely inheritable variety called Huntington's Disease (HD – also called Huntington's Chorea). If one parent has the disease, 50% of the offspring are at risk. A particularly unpleasant twist

[22] Jellinger KA. Very old onset parkinsonism: A clinical–pathological study. Parkinsonism Relat Disord. 2018 Jul 24. pii: S1353–8020(18)30326–2. doi: 10.1016/j.parkreldis.2018.07.015.

to its heritability is that HD doesn't usually become obvious until the sufferer is old enough to have produced children. There are now diagnostic and predictive tests for people and embryos at risk but many potential sufferers prefer not to know their diagnosis. Those who do want to know their own fate can also learn the genetic status of their potential offspring. Whether they are normally–conceived foetuses or embryos created by *in vitro* fertilisation, the affected ones can be identified *in utero* or before implantation and nearly all potential parents who undergo testing want the foetuses or embryos that carry the disease to be aborted, or not to be implanted.

That is not because – as with abortion for Down syndrome discussed in Chapter 15 – prospective parents fear that the offspring would prove to be difficult or challenging children with limited intellectual ability and potential for independence. HD can occasionally start causing problems in adolescence but most sufferers show no signs of disease until well after they have left home. During their adolescence, it is their affected father or mother who is likely to start causing problems or become overtly demented. Another feature that makes HD even nastier than Alzheimer's disease is its very slow onset and prolonged course, death typically occurring in the 50s or 60s, twenty years or more after its initial manifestations. Furthermore, HD is accompanied by increasingly obvious twitching and writhing ('chorea' shares the same Greek root as 'choreography') so that patients are not just demented but distressing to look at, especially for their offspring who know or fear that the same terrifying fate may befall them. In the circumstances, it is not surprising that there is a significantly increased incidence of unassisted suicide in identified HD patients, (nearly nine times greater than average[23]) usually when the disease is at a

---

relatively early stage.[24] The reasons for suicide presumably vary but a desire to avoid reaching the advanced stage of HD must surely be prominent. Although neurological symptoms like twitching are often the first sign and occur well before the dementia stage arrives, HD – just like Alzheimer's or other dementias – can also present as various mental disturbances, as discussed in Ch 3. If the family history of HD is not known, the underlying cause of the disturbed behaviour may not be recognized until later.

There are also some rare medical conditions that are not primarily brain diseases but can affect the brain as well as other organs. Despite their rarity, it is important for doctors to be aware of them because they can often be treated and the dementia they cause can be arrested or even reversed. (Dementia is a set of symptoms with several causes, not a specific disease.) That is why patients referred to a specialist clinic because of early or suspected dementia will have various blood tests done, as well as brain scans and precise (neuro)psychological tests of memory and brain function. The reversible causes include both benign and malignant brain tumours, especially slow-growing ones; syphilis; an underactive thyroid (hypothyroidism); vitamin B12 deficiency, typically associated with pernicious anaemia (an uncommon blood disorder) or a vegan diet; and Lyme Disease, which is due to chronic infection by a non–venereal cousin of the bacterium that causes syphilis.

Occasionally, a severe depressive illness may make a patient behave in ways that suggest early dementia. Conversely, the brain changes in early dementia may trigger a first episode of depression (or mania) in someone predisposed by family history to unipolar (usually depressive) or bipolar (manic–

---

[24] Di Maio L, Squitieri F, Napolitano G, Campanella G, Trofatter J, Conneally M. Suicide risk in Huntington's disease. J Med Genet 1993, 30; 293–5.

depressive) mood disorders. Brain damage from bleeding or blocked arteries, which would cause a typical stroke if it affected areas of the brain controlling movement or speech, can cause acute and often relatively brief confusional states if it affects other areas. I won't go into the reversible causes in detail but since GPI is now so rare that most psychiatrists practising in Britain will never have seen a case, and because it used to be both common and a theme of plays and novels in the days before syphilis became treatable, I give a brief account of the only patient with this condition that I had the good fortune – in terms of clinical experience – to treat. Dementia isn't a cheerful topic and a story with a happy ending will do no harm. I've put it at the end of the book as an Appendix for those who are interested.

I have grouped dementia into three approximate grades of severity – mild, moderate and severe. That is how it is often graded by clinicians and the grades are fairly obvious. Mild or 'early' dementia is the stage at which memory is clearly declining but something resembling normal life and employment may still be possible. Mental Capacity will nearly always be preserved and people who live alone may still be able to do so without danger to themselves or others. In 'moderate' dementia, paid work is usually no longer possible (though painters, poets, potters, dog-breeders and writers may continue for a while) and the social and leisure activities that previously enlivened normal life become progressively more difficult or impossible. It is also the stage in which Mental Capacity is likely to be lost. At some point in 'moderate' dementia, the question of daily home help, institutional care or sheltered living is likely to arise, especially if dementia is accompanied by other common degenerative diseases of old age affecting mobility, vision or hearing, which often happens. The need for nursing home admission or 24-hour home care typically arises about 3.5 years on average after an Alzheimer diagnosis and a little under two years for Lewy body dementia[25] At that stage, conversation of sorts may still be possible but the events of the previous day or even of earlier the same day are progressively more unlikely to feature in it. In severe or advanced dementia, any sort of conversational exchange becomes increasingly difficult or impossible, family members are usually unrecognized or misidentified and assistance with personal hygiene becomes steadily more essential. Mental Capacity cannot exist. This is usually the stage of incontinence and feeding difficulties. There is wide variation in the duration of the various stages of Alzheimer dementia but given an average diagnosis-to-death period of seven years, a rough guide could be summarized as 3-4 years each for the early and moderate stages and 1-2 years for the advanced stage.[26]

To add some detailed personal accounts of Alzheimer-type dementias to the cases I observed sporadically in clinical practice, I asked people who had been close to someone with dementia if they could provide brief pictures and timelines of its progression. They appear in Chapter 4.

---

[25] Rongve A, Vossius C, Nore S, Testad I, Aarsland D. Time until nursing home admission in people with mild dementia: comparison of dementia with Lewy bodies and Alzheimer's dementia. Int J Geriatr Psychiat. 2014 Apr;29(4):392–8. doi: 10.1002/gps.4015. Epub 2013 Aug 13.

[26] Komarova NL1, Thalhauser CJ. High degree of heterogeneity in Alzheimer's disease progression patterns. PLoS Comput Biol. 2011 Nov;7(11):e1002251. doi: 10.1371/journal.pcbi.1002251. Epub 2011 Nov 3.

3

Brain, Mind, Memory, Personhood and Identity in Dementia

The brain is by far the most complex organ in the body but after maintaining life by controlling breathing, pulse, blood pressure and other basic but vital tasks, its most important function is to process information from inside and outside our bodies. When the heart isn't working properly, it doesn't pump blood as it should. When the brain isn't working properly, it doesn't process information as it should and that shows itself in several ways that are not mutually exclusive. Although impaired short-term memory is the commonest early sign of Alzheimer dementia, it is not the only one, because physical and/or structural brain disease of any kind – from head injuries to cerebral tumours – increases the likelihood of all types of mental disturbance. As well as some memory loss, the main presenting symptoms of Frau Auguste Deter, who turned out – following the post mortem microscopic examination of her brain – to be Prof. Alois Alzheimer's first case of the disease that bears his name, were excessive jealousy and delusions of infidelity. She became ill in her 40s and died aged 56.[27] For some people, the damage to brain cells in the cerebral

---

[27] Alzheimer A. Uber eine eigenartige erkrankung der hirnrinde. Allgemeine Zeitschrift fur Psychiatrie und Psychisch–Gerichtliche Medizin. 1907; 64:146–148.

cortex that leads to dementia may be heralded by disturbances of mood – depression or its flip-side, mania – but anxiety, obsessional behaviour, hallucinations, loss of customary social inhibitions, delusions and personality change can also occur. In one case, the early symptoms of a woman who eventually turned out to have late onset Huntington's Disease were misdiagnosed for several years as being 'hysterical' in origin.[28] If they are severe and come out of the blue in a person aged 60 or over with no previous history of mental illness, such disturbances will probably lead to thorough physical investigations including a brain scan, though if the Alzheimer process is at a very early stage, the scans may be normal. However, if there have been previous episodes of depression or mania, for example, the latest episode may understandably be regarded as a recurrence or an exacerbation. Only if it fails to improve in the way that previous episodes improved may the diagnosis be reviewed and further investigations ordered.

Of course, 'depression' may be a normal and understandable reaction to memory problems, especially if tests indicate that they are the first signs of a dreaded and incurable illness. The same applies to consideration of deliverance from that fate. As the author Terry Pratchett put it in a BBC Dimbleby Lecture, "a person may make a decision to die because the balance of their mind is level, realistic, pragmatic, stoic and sharp. … In short, their minds may well be in better balance than the world around them."[29] It can take months to decide whether the depression is mainly 'understandable' or mainly due to some presumed (but still rather elusive) disturbance in brain chemistry and physiology. If it is due mainly to recent brain changes

---

[28] Nogueira JM, Franco AM, Mendes S, Valadas A, Semedo C, Jesus G. Huntington's Disease in a Patient Misdiagnosed as Conversion Disorder. Case Rep Psychiatry. 2018 Feb 18;2018:3915657. doi: 10.1155/2018/3915657. eCollection 2018.

[29] https://www.theguardian.com/society/2010/feb/02/terry-pratchett-assisted-suicide-tribunal

and is not a recurrence or reactivation of a true depressive or bipolar *illness*, it often fails to respond to antidepressants or other treatments, including psychological ones. A recent review noted that: "..the manifestations of [Alzheimer Dementia (AD)] are not limited to cognitive symptoms; rather, they include a range of neuropsychiatric symptoms (NPS) of AD. *The near universal prevalence of NPS in AD, combined with the serious and disabling effects they have on patients and caregivers, has focused significant recent attention on the fact that few effective and safe treatments exist".*[30] [my emphasis] It is probably fortunate that as dementia progresses and insight is lost, 'understandable' depression due to awareness of decline and the implications of the diagnosis tends to disappear. Often, it is replaced by apathy or agitation.[31] The most dramatic symptom of brain damage from disease or injury is an epileptic fit (or seizure). Fits are quite common following strokes, brain tumours and severe head injuries and although they are less common in dementia, the incidence is increased about five–fold compared with age–matched non–demented controls. There is some recent evidence that electrical disturbances typical of epilepsy – but not leading to visible seizures – occur in nearly half of dementia patients and that patients with these subclinical seizures suffer more rapid cognitive declines.[32] Its relevance, according to the authors, is that anti–epileptic medication may turn out to slow the decline.

---

[30] Geda YE, Schneider LS, Gitlin LN, et al. Neuropsychiatric symptoms in Alzheimer's disease: Past progress and anticipation of the future. Alzheimers Dement. 2013 September ; 9(5): 602–608. doi:10.1016/j.jalz.2012. 12.001.

[31] Harwood DG, Sultzer DL, Wheatley MV. Impaired insight in Alzheimer disease: association with cognitive deficits, psychiatric symptoms, and behavioral disturbances. Neuropsychiatry Neuropsychol Behav Neurol. 2000 Apr;13(2):83–8.

[32] Vossel KA, Ranasinghe KG, Beagle AJ, et al. Incidence and impact of subclinical epileptiform activity in Alzheimer's disease. Ann Neurol. 2016 Dec;80(6):858–870. doi: 10.1002/ana.24794. Epub 2016 Nov 7.

Just because dementia is due to an obvious brain disease doesn't make the disturbances in thought, perception and behaviour that it causes any less serious than those that are due to 'ordinary' depressive, bipolar or schizophrenia-like illnesses. Both dementia and schizophrenia are treated or managed by psychiatrists; they are not primarily cared for by the neurologists who specialize in brain diseases like Parkinsonism, multiple sclerosis or epilepsy that do not usually cause serious problems with cognition, perception or behaviour. When those 'neurological' brain diseases do cause psychoses, mood disorders or cognitive impairment, as all of them do in a proportion of cases, psychiatrists get involved and may take over most or all of their care. That is why these conditions – including dementia – are often called 'neuropsychiatric'.

Many dementia patients and their family members do not like to think of dementia as a mental or psychiatric illness, but definitions of mental illness or 'madness' revolve around behaviour, thought processes, perceptions, interactions with other people and personality, all of which are seriously impaired or altered as dementia progresses. The main difference is that most major mental illness first becomes apparent before the age of 30 and often makes lasting employment and relationships difficult or even impossible. (Of 1074 largely schizophrenic patients admitted – mostly in their 20s or early 30s – in North Wales over five decades around 1900, when marriage was the norm and divorce rare, 60% were unmarried.[33]) Despite much campaigning by psychiatrists and mental health advocates, that characteristic feature of severe mental illness – and the often imperfect response to treatment, especially in schizophrenia and personality disorders – understandably if regrettably leads

---

[33] Healy D, Le Noury J, Linden SC, et al. The incidence of admissions for schizophrenia and related psychoses in two cohorts: 1875e1924 and 1994e2010 BMJ Open 2012;2:e000447. doi:10.1136/bmjopen –2011–000447

to stigma. Dementia mostly affects people with no previous history of severe mental illness or stigma and while dementia attracts its own varieties of discrimination, in the early stages stigma is likely to be balanced by feelings of compassion, sympathy and regret that previously well–functioning and even admirable citizens have been struck down just when they should be enjoying retirement after exemplary or merely unremarkable lives. An entire philosophical cottage industry has grown up around the idea that Mad King George III wasn't *really* mad because he allegedly had porphyria and not a more plebeian, stigmatized and 'ordinary' condition like schizophrenia. Nevertheless – and there is no argument about this aspect of the story – George III was so disturbed, divorced from reality and incapable of sensible discussion that for varying periods starting quite early in his long reign, he was unable to do his rather important job; and not just a little bit unable but absolutely, totally unable. His problems were not that he was too weak, feverish, breathless or doubled up with pain to meet his ministers, discuss policy or sign documents and neither had he suffered a stroke that affected his speech or handwriting. In other words, they were not physical problems, so they must have been mental, psychiatric or behavioural problems, and serious ones at that. Furthermore, the physicians who treated him were not even called 'alienists' (a late 19th C term) or psychiatrists; they were called 'mad doctors'.

The porphyria theory may have been attractive to dramatists and paradoxically – despite its strong hereditary component – to monarchists but it has been comprehensively demolished. Even the famous 'blue urine' scene in the film version of Alan Bennett's play has been shown to be due to the incorrect deciphering of handwritten medical notes. No blue urine was ever recorded in them and in any case, the urine in porphyria turns reddish-brown, not blue. The 'Madness of George III' was almost certainly manic-depressive illness but his recurrent episodes of mania were overshadowed by probable Alzheimer dementia in his final decade.[34] Most of what we call schizophrenia and severe manic–depressive illness is also probably due to brain diseases. It's just that the diseases are more chemical and less well understood, at present, than the more obvious atrophic processes with visible tissue loss that cause dementia. The stigma attached to them arises mainly from their tendency to blight the whole of an adult life, rather than just the last few years of it.

Because we generally base our close and important relationships with other adults on the reasonable assumption that their personalities – agreeable or not – are fairly consistent and predictable, the changes in personality caused by dementia are often extremely disturbing and distressing. As a general rule, personality changes in early and moderate dementia tend towards exaggerated versions of the previous personality. Sweet-natured and kindly people may become – at least for a while – even more sweet–natured; argumentative and controlling ones may become even more controlling. That can be bad enough but sometimes, people who were always considerate of the feelings of others become very insensitive. At its most embarrassing, that can lead to unwanted and unwelcome sexual advances by both men and women. What the literature calls 'Inappropriate Sexual Behaviour" (ISB) is not rare.[35] While "the most likely change in the sexual behaviour of a person with dementia is indifference",[36] ISB becomes commoner in

---

[34] Peters T. King George III and the porphyria myth – causes, consequences and re–evaluation of his mental illness with computer diagnostics. Clin Med 2015 Vol 15, No 2: 168–72

[35] Perhaps this was what the waspish art critic Brian Sewell had in mind when he coined the phrase 'penile dementia'.

[36] Cipriani G, Ulivi M, Danti S, Lucetti C, Nuti A. Sexual disinhibition and dementia. Psychogeriatrics. 2016 Mar;16(2):145–53. doi: 10.1111/psyg.12143. Epub 2015 Jul 28.

the moderate and severe stages and may include hypersexuality, changes in sexual preference, paedophilia, promiscuity and marital infidelity.[37] In Sweden, 18% of a group of dementia patients had attracted the attention of the police.[38] However, the behavioural consequences of brain damage are unpredictable and very occasionally beneficial. A disturbed Canadian teenager who responded to his mother's exasperated cry 'why don't you just shoot yourself?' by actually doing so, survived the low-velocity bullet that traversed one of his frontal lobes. As a result of this DIY lobotomy, his behaviour greatly improved and his already high IQ increased after the disappearance of crippling obsessive–compulsive symptoms.[39]

When dementia causes major personality changes, important but complex problems of identity, personhood, philosophy, law and neuroscience arise when decisions have to be made about which personality – the old or the new – is to be given priority, most notably when following the instructions in a 'living will' (a phrase that I prefer and sometimes use here because it is still more widely used and understood than the officially favoured terms 'advance directive' or 'advance decision'). Two researchers describe "the hypothetical case of 'Margo', who made a living will, stating that she would wish to refuse treatment in the event of her becoming demented. However, despite, or perhaps because of, her dementia she now takes delight in small pleasures (e.g., peanut butter and jelly sandwiches). Margo might be said

---

[37] Abdo CH. Sexuality and couple intimacy in dementia. Curr Opin Psychiatry. 2013 Nov;26(6):593–8. doi: 10.1097/YCO.0b013e328365 a262.

[38] Liljegren M, Landqvist Waldö M, Rydbeck R, Englund E. Police Interactions Among Neuropathologically Confirmed Dementia Patients: Prevalence and Cause. Alzheimer Dis Assoc Disord. 2018 Aug 8. doi: 10.1097/WAD.0000000000000267.

[39] Solyom L, Turnbull IM, Wilensky M. A case of self–inflicted leucotomy. Brit J Psychiat 1987; 151: 855–7.

to be unaware that she has dementia, and is perhaps unaware of her previously stated preferences; however, she is aware of pleasure". Some ethicists argue that that "if we refuse the living will in these circumstances we are not being compassionate towards the whole person, the person who has tragically become demented". Others ask "whether we should deny to Margo the right that competent people have to change their mind?...The question then becomes whether we can treat the competent pre-demented Margo and her subsequent self as two different persons, the current 'person' being largely unaware of the former?"[40] Presumably, as Margot's dementia advanced and deprived her of mental capacity, her original instructions would resume their primacy but the hypothetical original Margot probably hoped that her life would end well before she got to the jelly and peanut butter stage.

Although the official title of the legal document is 'advance decision', the term 'living will' is particularly appropriate in this context – and more appropriate than the official alternatives – if we compare living wills with ordinary wills. In both cases, the will is usually made long before death becomes likely and when the person making the will (the *testator*) is still in reasonably good health. In both cases 'mental capacity' is assumed and though it is called 'testamentary capacity' in the case of an ordinary will, it is very similar. Both a living will and an ordinary will can be challenged if the testator is thought to have lacked capacity when the will was signed. The same applies to any subsequent alterations or codicils. In the case of ordinary wills, challenges are not infrequent when family members, who had expected to be among the beneficiaries, discover that a few months or even weeks before death, the

---

[40] Bennett R, Harris J. Dementia and end of life decisions. In J. O'Brien, D. Ames, & A. Burns (Eds.), Dementia (2nd edition) 2000. London: Arnold. 279–281

testator had altered the will in favour of a carer or someone who had only recently befriended the testator (or that the testator had given all her estate to a cats' home). If a testator suffers from dementia, any alterations that were made when capacity had clearly been lost are invalid in the case of an ordinary will and it is difficult to see why the same principles should not apply to living wills as well. They include the principle that the choices and decisions of the intact, consistent, pre-dementia, capacity-possessing personality of the testator take absolute precedence over any choices and decisions of the recently-altered, severely brain-damaged, capacity-lacking personality that is the consequence of even moderately advanced dementia.

While non-demented adult patients have a fairly general and presumptive right, in many jurisdictions, to see their medical notes and to know the truth about their condition if they want it, that right is often not accepted in dementia. Even in the early stages, information may be withheld, filtered or euphemized. "Although findings vary from study to study, the following points emerge: People with dementia are less often told the diagnosis than are family members [and] are given euphemisms − 'memory loss' − more often than family members, [who] would often prefer the person not to be told, despite agreeing they would want to know if they were in that situation. [They] feel the person will be distressed by the information and (perhaps paradoxically) that the person will not understand anyway." However, "People with dementia who have been told the diagnosis generally feel this is preferable even though a proportion find it upsetting".[41] The same authors found that "Lies may be seen as being less important in people who are unaware of what is happening anyway". Among

---

[41] Woods B, Pratt R. Awareness in dementia: ethical and legal issues in relation to people with dementia. Aging Ment Health. 2005 Sep;9(5):423–9.

staff working in care facilities, "96% admitted having lied to residents, most commonly to ease residents' distress (88% of respondents). However, 40% of staff reported using lies to gain the person's compliance with treatment and 28% and 36% to get the person to do something and simply to save time, respectively. Most staff recognized that lies could also cause complications, as well as solve problems". The authors add, though, that "selective truth-telling is, of course, a common strategy in every sphere of life".

4

What Dementia Looks Like

Impaired memory for recent events is the commonest change that makes people wonder if they have a real problem rather than what is usually called 'benign' or 'mild cognitive impairment' (MCI). That sort of 'now what was it that I went upstairs for?' forgetfulness is common once we get past 60 and even if it becomes more noticeable, it will not necessarily progress to Alzheimer's, but it does so in getting on for 50% of cases, depending in part on what specific areas of cognition are found to be impaired on detailed testing. The typical interval between first noticing memory impairment and having a diagnosis of dementia confirmed is about three years for Alzheimer's.[42] Often, the memory impairment is first noticed by family members or friends. This may be more likely if the degenerative process affects the frontal lobes early in the disease, with a consequent early loss of insight or concern. The fronto–temporal and Lewy body dementias may progress more rapidly than Alzheimer dementia and are also more likely to start

---

[42] Bature F, Guinn BA, Pang D, Pappas Y. Signs and symptoms preceding the diagnosis of Alzheimer's disease: a systematic scoping review of literature from 1937 to 2016. BMJ Open. 2017 Aug 28;7(8):e015746. doi: 10.1136/bmjopen–2016–015746.

before the age of 65 – which was regarded as the cutoff point for what we used to call 'pre–senile' dementia. Fortunately, with the exception of Huntington's disease, it is uncommon for any sort of dementia to begin before the late 50s. Only around 3% of people will develop Alzheimer dementia before reaching 65 (vascular dementia is also uncommon before 65) but the Alzheimer risk rises steadily with age. At 75, it is still less than 10% but after 75, the risk rises steeply. By 85 – by which time many patients may also have other chronic illnesses affecting both mobility and quality of life – about a third of people will have developed it and by 95, about half.

This chapter is a collection of real case-histories of people with dementia as seen not by doctors, nurses or researchers but by their carers, their partners or observant acquaintances who are non-demented residents of care homes. All names are fictitious except for Robert, whose story is an expanded version of an account published on the website of an Australian dementia organization.[43] I am grateful to Robert's partner Gary for adding more details and to the other informants for their stories.

GEORGE

George was the father of a GP on the south coast of England. The course of his Alzheimer's was relatively short – five years from onset to death – though he might have lived for another year or more if an acute illness had not intervened. Despite being in an advanced state of dementia, he was moved from a nursing home to a hospital in his last days and active surgical intervention was considered even though if he had survived the surgery, he would almost certainly have ended up with even less awareness and an even poorer quality of life.

---

[43] https://www.dementiadaily.org.au/gary-and-robert/

"When he was 84, five years before he died, my father's cognitive function was still unimpaired. At that time, following my younger brother's death, he had dealt with all the legal matters and probate but some six months later, my mother began to report erratic driving and short temper with some forgetfulness. He would pull out without looking in the driving mirror but the first thing we could not avoid recognising and accepting as dementia was when my 65-year-old Australian cousin made his first ever visit to the UK and stayed with my parents. Dad went to drive him and his wife to Poole Quay. He could not remember the way and abandoned the attempt but managed to find his way home.

He began to stop showering or even shaving and personal hygiene became a battleground between him and my mother. We took away his car keys and arranged an assessment after his GP tested him with the MMSE [The Mini Mental State Examination is a standard short screening test for dementia] and found that his score had fallen sharply in the space of six months. At the initial consultation with the memory clinic psychiatrist, he made jokes to hide his memory loss. Before we went in I asked him his age and he said '67', but he was 85. I asked him who was the last Prime Minister that he could recall. He said 'Clement Atlee' [1945–50] but when the laughter was over I pressed him and it was actually Edward Heath [1970–74]. He couldn't even spontaneously recall the sainted Margaret Thatcher. (I remember reading that she ruined one of the standard memory questions because people with quite severe memory loss often remembered her name, even when they had forgotten most other things.) The psychiatrist agreed with our decision to prevent him from driving but Dad's anger about this went on for another year.

By the time he was 87, his physical decline was quite marked. He had difficulty walking more than fifty paces, due to peripheral neuropathy affecting his feet and lower legs.

No cause was ever found. A couple of years before the dementia appeared, he had an episode of acute heart failure, from which he was saved by triple coronary artery stents. His feet were always the limiting factor after the stenting; never his heart,.

At 87, he also began to experience falls on the stairs and they moved into a flat, spending four months living with us while their house was sold. Before the dementia began, he had tried for many years to persuade my mother to move into a flat but now he didn't want to leave the house at all. I asked him why. He paused and thought long and hard before replying (with great prescience and insight) 'I think I am worried that if I leave here, I will never know quite where I am again'.

His last eight months were spent in the flat, which was opposite the entrance to Poole Harbour, a place he had always loved. Each night he would ask my mother if they were going home, because he thought he was on holiday on the Isle of Wight and that he was looking at the Solent. (We had holidayed there in 1964). He did not recall where Sandbanks was [it's a famously up-market harbour–front area] and didn't know he was in Poole, despite having lived there since 1970 – the Edward Heath era indeed. He avoided friends because he didn't know or recognise anyone and this embarrassed him. The company he most sought and enjoyed was Toby, our Jack Russell terrier. Toby would simply light up when he appeared and go over to him for the back massage that he knew only Dad could do properly. And of course Dad knew that Toby would ask no awkward questions.

Despite increasing assistance from visiting care staff, he eventually became unmanageable in the flat and was admitted to a care home. Two days later, he fell and sustained a subarachnoid [brain] haemorrhage, and was transferred to hospital. Despite his very advanced dementia, it seems that the hospital doctors seriously considered operating on his brain. Fortunately, the neurosurgeons advised against it. During his last seven days, he was on a drip that contained midazolam [a Valium-type sedative which is also – perhaps unnecessarily in this case – a powerful amnesic agent] and diamorphine [pharmaceutical quality heroin] a powerful analgesic and respiratory depressant, presumably with the unstated intention of ensuring that his death occurred sooner rather than later. However, until near the end, he was not completely unresponsive. The mention of Toby's name would bring a smile to his face, even when his eyes were shut and he could not speak. I wish I had smuggled Toby in for a last goodbye. But I didn't."

ANDREW

Andrew's story was supplied by his daughter. He was one of the first Alzheimer patients for whom I did a psychiatric and mental capacity assessment after he applied to Dignitas. Although by that time he had definite cognitive impairment and the diagnosis was not in doubt, he still scored 27/30 on the MMSE. This reinforces the advice later in the book that a referral for full assessment at a memory clinic should be requested – by the patient, the family or the GP – as soon as consistent memory problems or other worrying symptoms appear. More elaborate neuropsychological tests measure particular areas of cognition and memory and make the results of subsequent tests easier to compare. Andrew's case also shows the difficulty of confident diagnosis in the early stages of Alzheimer's, the understandable tendency to diagnose 'depression' in the hope that antidepressants will help over and above their considerable placebo effects, and the need to distinguish between depression as a *brain illness* (which might conceivably respond to antidepressants in some cases) and depression as an *understandable reaction to progressive impairment and an Alzheimer diagnosis* (which is rather unlikely to respond to medication except at a placebo level). As a rule, that sort of depressive reaction to Alzheimer's can at most be only modestly and temporarily alleviated by counselling. Significantly, it was only getting accepted by Dignitas that lastingly improved Andrew's mood.

"The first sign of change in Dad was a very gradual loss of confidence along with increasingly frequent forgetful incidents, which in retrospect probably started several years before he was diagnosed with Alzheimer's. Over this time my Mum sometimes told me that she thought there was something wrong but I just didn't believe her. Maybe I was in denial, and I certainly knew nothing at all about Alzheimer's at the time, but I couldn't see any major worrying changes. Dad and I still enjoyed in-depth discussions about all sort of issues and had a very satisfying relationship. In late 2010 my parents went on a long term trip abroad and during this time it became apparent that Dad wasn't able to hold enough information to play bridge any more, something that he'd always enjoyed. He was also beginning to forget some of the key biological facts that he'd known and taught all though his life and started having some panic attacks and confusion. Dad and Mum were concerned enough for Dad to see a doctor and have a brain scan after which the doctor told Dad that he had mild cognitive impairment and there was nothing to worry about.

On his return to the UK in the summer of 2011, Dad could no longer manage his financial affairs and other administrative issues. This was a major change and very difficult for him to face as he'd been very organised and competent all his life. His driving had become increasingly erratic and he very reluctantly decided to stop driving. He visited his GP and was referred to the Memory Clinic who said that he was suffering from depression. Both Mum and Dad were very doubtful about this diagnosis but two further appointments at the Memory Clinic confirmed the diagnosis and Dad was prescribed antidepressants, which he reluctantly took. Over this time he became less and less able to take part in the things he enjoyed. He'd always been a keen cook and had to stop cooking, he started putting things away in very odd places and was surprised when they were found, wondering how they could have got there. He had been a botanist and had always loved nature and studying plants but he was no longer able to do this. He began to find it difficult to read and started using a piece of card to move down the page of text as he read as he found it difficult to move from the end of one line to the beginning of the next line.

He began to get confused about where his friends lived in the block of flats he lived in and also finding my house when he came to visit me. He began to become disorientated when he was out and found it difficult to find his way back home. Eventually he was unable to find his way from his home to my home, a short route that he had travelled many times. Occasionally he said that he didn't recognise his own home. He became unable to dress himself and shower himself and eventually had to stop reading entirely. At this stage the only thing he could do that brought him some pleasure was listening to story tapes, which he enjoyed as long as the story line was fairly simple. Even at this stage he was still able to have interesting and rational conversations and people who met him often commented that they couldn't believe that he had Alzheimer's disease. In October 2012 a consultant geriatric psychiatrist visited him in his home and spent an hour really listening to him and his concerns and finally diagnosed him with Alzheimer's. Alongside the intense sadness that we all felt, there was also a sense of relief that there was explanation for his difficulties. He died two years later at Dignitas. When he got the 'green light' he was so happy, finally able to fully relax in the knowledge that he could have the release that he wanted."

ROBERT

In contrast to the cases above with a fairly short trajectory, Robert's twelve years between onset and death are relatively unusual, though certainly not rare. It also reminds us that with hindsight, early signs of dementia can often be recognised several years before it becomes obvious. He was the first of my contemporaries – and so far, the only one – to get Alzheimer's. Never send to know for whom the bell tolls....

Robert – a barrister among other talents – was 64 when he met Gary, who was 48. By that time, he had retired from the bar and lived mainly on income from property investments. As well as being a friend, he had retained me as an expert witness in some of his court cases and I knew him quite well but I didn't see much of him around that time because he had been working and living abroad. With hindsight, Gary thinks Robert's dementia had already started to affect him because although they arranged to meet for lunch the day after their first encounter, Robert had forgotten until he phoned him. Despite this poor start, it became a close relationship. Robert was very good company and Gary carried on working. He was very fond of Robert and thought his occasional lapses of memory were just ordinary 'senior moments'. It was another two years before a visitor who hadn't seen Robert for several years noticed both that he was forgetful and that he seemed to be frequently checking the date on the telephone handset. The penny dropped and Gary persuaded Robert to see his GP, who referred him to a memory clinic but it was another two years before the specialist told him that Robert had Alzheimer dementia. Because Gary was 'only' his partner, he had to ask repeatedly for the information. By this stage, he did not recognize me when I visited but had become quite skilled at disguising his deficits.

Robert had always kept a daily journal but a year later, when he was 69, he stopped writing and never resumed it.

Around that time, he started to forget his PIN number and his normally free and amusing conversation became progressively more limited but he continued to take daily walks and he could manage unaccompanied journeys by public transport if the route was familiar. Three years later at 72, he no longer initiated conversation and gave only brief replies. Robert had never been a heavy drinker but his walks now regularly included a visit to his local pub, where his shrinking brain meant that even small amounts of alcohol could make him unsteady. Often he seemed to forget that he had already had a few drinks. The staff kept an eye on him but they sometimes had to call an ambulance after a fall. Gary was now finding it very difficult to combine his work with being an increasingly full-time carer. He gave up his job, rented out his flat and moved from Britain with Robert to a single-storey property that Robert owned in an Australian country town.

In that year, Robert began to be incontinent of urine. A relatively benign and slow-growing prostate cancer was diagnosed and responded to hormonal treatment but within a few months, he became doubly incontinent. The local social services offered 16 hours of respite care per week and the incontinence pads they provided were generally effective but at times Gary had to change the bedclothes (and Robert) daily. By the end of that year – the ninth – Robert started to forget who Gary was and he sometimes became violent when he tried to undress him for his shower. Occasionally, Gary instinctively hit back – something that made him very remorseful. That was one of the things that made him seek some counselling, as was the fact that he 'hated having to micro–manage him', though he never had more than monthly sessions.

During year ten, it became necessary to lock him into the house. After another 18 months, he was admitted to a nursing home where, as Gary described it, he treated him 'as if I were just another member of the staff'. Robert's appetite remained good, though most of his food needed to be liquidized. He survived for another year and was bed-ridden for his final two months, during which he developed a few bedsores. It was 11 years from the first referral for probable Alzheimer's until his death and 13 years from what were probably the first signs. That is almost twice as long as the average for Alzheimer dementia but far from uncommon. It's a lot less than the average for Huntington dementia.

A prominent feature of Robert's case was his almost complete lack of insight. He never admitted or even mentioned the diagnosis and Gary thinks that underneath the bland exterior, he was scared. That might be so but though I never saw his brain scans, I suspect that frontal lobe atrophy was an even more important factor. I knew Robert's views on most topics and although I don't recall any specific conversations about deliverance, it is unlikely that we never discussed it, especially since his mother had been the matron of a care home and Robert looked after her when she became blind. I am sure that he knew my views and I am equally sure that he never expressed any personal or general opposition to them. This is further evidence of the need to make dementia-specific living wills well before dementia starts to become increasingly common after we hit 60. Many people with early dementia retain sufficient insight into their diagnosis to consider their options but many do not. Gary had no doubts about what he would do if he developed early Alzheimer's. 'I'd definitely be off to Switzerland'.

The four following case-histories were recorded by friends of mine who live in private or charitable retirement homes in Britain, where the residents had all previously been employed in professional and managerial jobs. Most of the cases involve patients who seem – for the moment - to be relatively happy most of the time despite their dementia but this happiness is not always shared by their family, friends or fellow-residents.

Furthermore, they are all in the early or moderate stages of dementia and – with one exception – will inevitably progress, if they live long enough, to a stage where they will almost certainly lose that happiness and even more certainly cause much unhappiness to those who love them and care for them.

PAULINE

Pauline (diagnosed with Alzheimer's four years ago) is a happy, attractive person. Now in her early 80s she lives in sheltered housing, with carers coming in four times a day. She is much loved by her friends and neighbours there, who knew her before dementia set in. She was a capable woman, wife of a high-ranking officer accustomed to entertaining and also doing valuable voluntary work.

The fact that she was a good and much loved mother is borne out by the regular and frequent visits from her daughters, holidays spent with them and trips out to lunch. She has difficulty remembering her daughters' names, is sometimes aware that one of them lives abroad but can't recall the name of the country. Pauline's loss of short-term memory led to marked increase in her alcohol consumption. She would go to the clubhouse bar and buy a bottle of wine, take it home and drink it, then after lunch and a snooze in her armchair, wake and consume another bottle in the early evening. She seemed to function perfectly well, reading the newspaper (though with no memory of what she read) and always watching the television news.

The carers make sure she manages personal hygiene and help with selecting her clothes each day, arranging hair and chiropody appointments etc. She always looks well-groomed and attractive and lunches in the dining room of the complex where she lives. Her tendency to break into cheerful song is a delight to many fellow diners but an embarrassment and annoyance to a few. Complimented one day on her outfit and hairdo, she put her hands to her head. "Good gracious, whatever have they done to me?" No memory at all of the morning's trip to the hairdresser. Pauline's sunny disposition cloaks her anxiety. "Dear me, what I doing here? Where am I going?" She has formed a close bond with her regular carers, treats them with respect and affection and is never irritable, aggressive or rude.

JENNIFER

Jennifer is a diminutive woman in her nineties. She worked in senior management in social services until she officially retired, then took on another full-time job until she finally retired in good health a decade or so later. She had never been seriously ill or spent time in hospital. Two years ago, she had a heart attack at home but didn't call an ambulance until she had had her weekly coiffure. Though instructed to lead a quieter life, she found this impossible and was soon back to her "gallivanting", visiting friends, serving on committees, keeping up with her large family, visiting museums, art galleries, historic houses and eating out in pubs and restaurants.

About four years ago, friends noticed that while Jennifer attempted to keep up the same frenetic pace, she was becoming more forgetful and increasingly confused – frequently losing or misplacing hat, gloves, coat, umbrella, her diary and all the little pieces of paper tucked into it. Missed engagements and double bookings resulted. Always an avid writer of letters and cards, this became an obsession. Multiple cards would be received for birthdays and Christmas; email messages would be sent 20 to 30 minutes apart, differently worded but containing the same information

Jennifer was given an inhaler for breathing difficulties but couldn't remember how to use it, despite being shown repeatedly and patiently. This led to her dialling 999 for an ambulance on seven nights over a two-week period. After that, it was decided that she should move in to a care home where there would always be someone on call at night. More lessons with the inhaler were given but some nights, she becomes frightened and rings for help several times.

Despite this, she continues to get out and about, bombards friends with requests to sign her out and accompany her on outings, disregards advice and blatantly breaks the rules of her care home. Conversation can be difficult as her short-term memory deteriorates further and her kind enquiries about one's family are repeated again and again until she can be distracted to talk about events in the past.

The next case is rather unusual and involves dementia – almost certainly due to a stroke mainly affecting parts of the brain not primarily concerned with movement or speech – that had a sudden onset but has not progressed much since then.

JOE

Joe, an 83-year-old retired architect, recently celebrated his diamond wedding anniversary. This was only a matter of weeks after he developed sudden onset dementia. The first sign appeared when, watching television with his wife and one of their daughters, he suddenly stood up with his back to the TV set and started walking round and round the room, not speaking, eyes blank, unresponsive to his wife and daughter. Consequent problems have included sleeplessness, inappropriate language and touching, urinating in the waste paper basket and not knowing how to operate the bathroom taps.

Formerly a gentle, kindly, talkative man, he has become more insistent and abrupt on the occasions when he speaks. The sleeping pills he has been prescribed ensure that his wife is able to get some rest at night. Joe spent a short period in respite care so that his wife - also more than 80 - could have a break. His erratic behaviour meant that he could not safely be left at home alone. Even the weekly shopping trip became a nightmare as he kept disappearing in the large supermarket.

In the care home dining room, his tendency to disruptive behaviour unsettles other residents, though he seems perfectly content to be there. Since going home, his behaviour has improved but his wife feels that she lives "walking on eggshells....Before, he was reliable; now he is unpredictable". There are good days and bad days.

Since the onset of dementia, Joe has lost a lot of weight and is increasingly unsteady on his feet. He still has a lovely smile and will greet friends by name when in speaking mood. On a recent visit to his rather severe female GP, he addressed her as "darling" – completely out of character and greatly surprising her. The strain of caring for a spouse with dementia is telling on his wife, though they have a loving family, whose members help as and when able. The sudden onset of Joe's dementia struck a cruel blow to this affectionate couple's old age. Once there was closeness and content; now a sense of unease exists. If Joe avoids further strokes with the help of appropriate medication, his behaviour may not change much but the longer he survives, the greater the risk that he may also develop an Alzheimer-type dementia that will progressively add to his existing brain damage. Since he went straight from normal brain function to a state of moderate dementia without passing through an early stage, he may well have lost the necessary insight for drawing-up a detailed living will and the mental capacity for contemplating or requesting MAID in Switzerland, if he was ever minded to do so.

The last case describes the kind of sexual disinhibition and inappropriate sexual behaviour that not infrequently occurs in dementia, especially when damage affects the frontal lobes, which have an important role in mediating social behaviour and impulse control.

MARK

Mark – an urbane, still handsome man in his late 70s who has travelled extensively and spent much of his life working abroad – now has Alzheimer's and lives in supported accommodation but likes to drink and socialise in the clubhouse bar. He has a girl-friend who comes to stay on occasions – a good-looking woman, probably in her mid-60s. They obviously enjoy a sexual relationship and he is relaxed and happy in her company.

One summer evening, he hammered on a neighbour's door, walked in and asked: "Are you the woman who invited me in for drinks this evening?" She said he was mistaken. He explained that someone had invited him and he couldn't remember who it was. Sent packing, he knocked on the doors of several other women living in the block. Ten minutes later he was back at his original port of call, barging in without knocking and waving a half-full bottle of wine. "Are you sure you didn't invite me?" She asked him to describe the woman who issued the invitation – tall, short, fat, thin, dark, fair? – but he had no idea. Asked where he was at the time of the invitation, he replied that he was in the shower. "I had to wrap a towel round me." This second time, he was hard to dislodge but left, plainly annoyed, to continue his search for the invisible woman.

A few minutes later he was back again and the mood had changed. The first visit, he had been full of charm; the second he was growing more insistent; by the third he was showing annoyance bordering on aggression. "I know it was you and that you want to have a drink with me." He tried to sit down but was ushered out very firmly and this time the door was locked behind him. Mark liked to display himself, naked, in front of his first-floor bedroom window. This gave the lady living opposite a shock when she opened her window. "Not a pretty sight" she reported. Adding to the spectacle was a pair of Mark's underpants hanging from a coat-hanger outside his window. As another resident remarked; "it's not what you expect in a historic Grade 1 listed building".

5

What Dementia Feels Like

Dementia, especially Alzheimer dementia, is the focus of large and increasing amounts of research into its causes, genetics, clinical features, brain changes, prognosis and treatment. Every day on average, at least ten new research papers appear on Medline if you search under 'Alzheimer'. However, all this information "stands in counterpoint to the lack of systematic inquiry around the lived experiences" of people with the condition.[44] Other researchers noted that "the number of studies dealing with the experiences of having and coping with dementia as expressed by the sufferers themselves has increased relatively slowly". Their paper begins forthrightly: "Among the general public there is a deep fear of developing dementia, which has led to an increasing number of people 'at risk' seeking ways (such as advance directives) to avoid undergoing progressive mental decline. The views of people with dementia are vital in obtaining a real answer to the question of how the disease affects people's lives and whether it actually involves

---

[44] McQuarrie CR. Experiences in early stage Alzheimer's disease: understanding the paradox of acceptance and denial. Aging Ment Health. 2005 Sep;9(5):430–41.

the suffering that so many fear." The authors, Marike de Boer and her colleagues – specializing in 'nursing home medicine' and Alzheimer's – looked at publications "describing aspects of dementia from the patient's perspective in the form of quotations, i.e. 'as told by the dementia sufferers themselves'."[45] Since people with dementia are human and therefore have a variety of backgrounds, personalities and personal philosophies, it is unsurprising that they experience dementia and respond to it in equally varied ways; at least until their failing brains make the expression of any views difficult or impossible.

In early dementia, these varied manifestations probably reflect a mixture of personality, domestic and philosophical factors, on the one hand, and brain changes on the other. Later on, as personalities, domestic relationships and existential concerns are progressively annihilated by the disease, the brain takes over. Some people are by nature optimists. "I do not like to think or speak of anything unpleasant", wrote the Rev. Joseph Priestley, the laid-back 18th century clergyman and discoverer of oxygen (and soda water). "I confide [i.e. believe, trust] in a good Providence, and generally look on the bright side of everything". He seems to have many modern followers. "I could be a lot worse" one Alzheimer patient commented. "This must be normal, I guess, for my age" said another. However, some respondents saw very clearly what lay ahead and were already alarmed by the changes they had noticed. "I'm losing my mind, my ability to know what's going on. I want to observe and feel part of life". "There is nothing left when you lose your mind". "Not being able to do anything... I don't want to lose everything".

The patient who responded (or retorted) "No, I don't have any trouble with my memory. Other people might have trouble

---

[45] de Boer M, Hertogh C, Dröes R–M, et al. Suffering from dementia – the patient's perspective: a review of the literature. *International Psychogeriatrics* (2007),19:6,1021–1039

with my memory but as far as I am concerned, Alzheimer's is not bothering me at all", might just have been expressing a natural cussedness and independence – the Alzheimer equivalent of "Don't shout at me. I'm not deaf". Alternatively, he might have been consciously or unconsciously using one of our oldest and commonest ways of dealing with bad news: denial. He might, though, have been demonstrating one of the symptoms of dementia that – depending on your point of view – is either one of its saving graces or one of its most worrying features: the progressive loss of insight that makes patients increasingly unable to recognise that their brain is failing and that they will eventually have nothing to say about anything. We met some examples in the previous chapter. Cussedness and independence will often yield to reality. So, though perhaps less often, does denial but when loss of insight is due to the loss of the part of the brain that is crucial for insight, it cannot be regained. However, the rate of loss is rather variable. A British 20-month follow up of 101 patients with early dementia concluded: "At least in the earlier stages of dementia, it should not be assumed that awareness will inevitably decrease as dementia progresses".[46] A US study of patients with both early and more advanced dementia warned that "even those with severe cognitive impairments can poignantly describe their feelings about having dementia."[47] That study, subtitled "View from inside", tried to identify the themes that emerged when 56 patients were asked the single question: "How have things been going for you lately?". It is an indication of how disabling dementia is

---

[46] Clare L, Nelis SM, Martyr A, Whitaker CJ, Marková IS, Roth I, Woods RT, Morris RG. Longitudinal trajectories of awareness in early–stage dementia. Alzheimer Dis Assoc Disord. 2012 Apr–Jun;26(2):140–7. doi: 10.1097/WAD.0b013e31822c55c4.

[47] Ostwald SK, Duggleby W, Hepburn KW. The stress of dementia: view from the inside. Am J Alzheimers Dis Other Demen. 2002 Sep–Oct;17(5):303–12.

that six of them could not respond with anything that could qualify as a 'theme', as exemplified in the following exchange:

Interviewer: How are things going for you?

Patient: How are things going for you . .
two . . . four . . . six . . . yeah.

All were still living "in the community" (i.e. presumably at home rather than in an institution) and most were white and had completed at least secondary education. Their mean age was 77.6 (range 47 to 97) and just over half were men. For 92%, 'loss' was the main theme. "They described loss of ability to initiate a conversation, loss of memory, loss of ability to think clearly, loss of contact with reality (i.e., hallucinations), loss of control over their environment and possessions, and loss of purpose in life."

Patients with hallucinations described a very typical and distressing frustration with people who didn't share their perceptions of reality. "I know they talked about me, about that…and I called the cops [but] when people know you are watching for them, they hide, you know…I didn't like people to talk that way 'cause I'm not hallucinating."

Nearly a third of patients talked about death. Some hoped they could live longer but most were concerned about the quality of their remaining life and the effect of dementia on their families. "Probably about all I can hope for is to have an easy death…I guess nobody can promise me that either [laughs] . . . except euthanasia, possibly." One man made it clear that he wanted his wife to be free to start another relationship. "I don't want her tied up…. I'd just as soon drown myself than live like that." Instead of the apparent apathy and withdrawal that are typical of more advanced dementia (when it is not causing frightening delusions and hallucinations) many of the people in this study appear to have experienced dementia as stressful.

Some patients with serious cognitive impairment on standard cognitive assessment scales such as the Mini Mental State Examination (MMSE) retained insight into their diagnosis. Reduced social contact worried some while others welcomed it because it reduced demands on their failing abilities. Reading eventually became impossible. When misidentifications and hallucinations did not make it difficult or impossible, family support was important and appreciated.

One personal account of Alzheimer's is particularly noteworthy in that it was written by a neurologist and also because he describes some very early symptoms.[48] When he was 55, Daniel Gibbs began to notice difficulty in recognising subtle smells. He did not know it at the time but this is a common feature of early Alzheimer's and may help to distinguish Mild Cognitive Impairment from more serious disturbances of memory.[49] At 60, after some genealogical researches, he accidentally discovered that he had an increased genetic risk of developing Alzheimer's. (see Chapter 12 for a more detailed discussion of Alzheimer genetics) but did not notice any memory disturbance until a year later. After another year, he retired from practice but volunteered to take part in several research and educational projects. He feels that knowing his diagnosis so early in the disease was helpful and it certainly motivated him to make sure all his financial affairs were in order and that his Durable Power of Attorney included "detailed instructions about end-of-life issues". He has made a few lifestyle changes, presumably takes medication that can slow the progress of dementia and still leads an active life. At 67, his dementia is still in the early

---

[48] Gibbs DM. Early awareness of Alzheimer disease: a neurologist's personal perspective. JAMA Neurol. 2019 Feb 18. doi: 10.1001/jamaneurol.2018.4910

[49] Devanand DP. Olfactory identification deficits, cognitive decline, and dementia in older adults. Am J Geriatr Psychiatry. 2016 Dec;24(12):1151-1157. doi: 10.1016/j.jagp.2016.08.010.

stage. Although he misses his work, "early stage [Alzheimer] has not been that bad and I am hoping for another five or ten years before entering the late stage". In his neurology clinic, he used to "avoid giving a firm [dementia] diagnosis at all costs" but now feels that this attitude is wrong. This reinforces my repeated advice that people should get a referral to a memory clinic if they or – as is more often the case – their family and friends notice memory problems that may (but also may not) be an early sign of dementia.

ALEX

To see and hear a person with early Alzheimer's instead of reading about one, you can access a local radio podcast[50] and a short YouTube documentary[51] featuring Alex Pandolfo. Alex is a 65-year old lecturer in law, sociology and psychology who arrived in academia via trades union activity as a bus driver and Oxford degrees at Ruskin and Nuffield Colleges. A proud Lancastrian and Manchester City supporter, he is a large, cheerful man with firm socialist views who is determined to make the best of his remaining days and to do as much as he can for the deliverance debate before he goes to Switzerland. He first noticed cognitive problems in his late 50s when marking dissertations, though he quips that some of them were just badly written. Having nursed his father through dementia, he knows exactly what lies in store – 'a life of misery, abuse and upsetting others'. His facebook group - The Right To Die With Dignity UK - has around 2000 members and organises live conferences. As discussed in Ch. 12, Alex's presumably high intelligence and 'cognitive reserve' may partly explain why the

---

[50] https://www.dropbox.com/s/mkhyhe4rjxxk02w/Thurnham%20
Mews%20Thurnham%20Street.m4a?dl=0

[51] https://www.youtube.com/watch?v=_E9gMT5pjE0

progress of his disease is relatively slow, even though early-onset Alzheimer's can progress more quickly. You can also see Alex's account of the response of the memory clinic psychiatrist when he mentioned Switzerland and deliverance.[52] He already suffered from several quite serious illnesses which, though treatable, would probably cause severe impairment of his quality of life eventually and he said that the Alzheimer diagnosis was just one additional reason why he might opt for assisted suicide. The psychiatrist's immediate response was that Alex must be suffering from 'depression' and he wanted to treat this 'illness' with antidepressants before treating the dementia, since there could be problems if antidepressants and anti-Alzheimer medication were prescribed simultaneously. Alex managed to persuade him to reverse his priorities but I am shocked – though not surprised – at the implication *by a psychiatrist* that anyone who is interested in alternatives to waiting for Nature to take its course must have an 'illness', rather than having an existential view that is broadly shared by over 80% of British citizens. It is really a psychiatric version of the Vatican's position (and until recently, the Church of England's position) that suicides can escape the damnation or excommunication that their grievous sin still officially deserves because all of them are presumed to be so insane that they were not responsible for their actions. I discuss it in more detail in Chapter 8 but as long ago as 1893, a Lancet editorial protested: "For a jury to return a verdict imparting insanity to a man without any evidence beyond the bare fact of suicide is an unworthy evasion."[53]

To end this chapter, here is a letter composed by a person with early dementia shortly before leaving for deliverance in Switzerland. I did the Mental Capacity assessment and

---

[52] https://www.facebook.com/100012302467462/videos/626625454 424198/

[53] Editorial, The legal fiction of the insanity of suicides. Lancet1893. 972.

the patient's family very kindly allowed me to publish this anonymised extract.

"...my memory is just slipping away from me now – in the face of that I feel helpless. So, I must write this down immediately – I want to go to LifeCircle in 5 days, or is it 4, for a MAS [Medically Assisted Suicide]. Nothing is more certain in my mind, and I don't want this dreadful loss of short term memory to get in the way, as seems the danger now. I MUST GO! That is my big fear – to finally lose memory altogether and to stop me going.

Apart from this very important thing, I would not want to leave you all. I love you all so dearly. I am sorry to be going, but I must go, because of my rapid memory loss.

I LOVE YOU ALL. I did intend to record my feelings every day, but I was too busy enjoying the last days!!!

So glad finally, I have put all this down on paper...I feel sure, and funnily enough excited! My life coming to a close, just at the right time. I am TIRED, very tired. I am not afraid."

[handwritten annotation: NO FEEDING ME FOR ME TO BE IN A DEMENTED STATE (OR PROBABLY OTHERWISE)]

6

Will You Still Need Me, Will You Tube-Feed Me, When I'm Ninety-Four?

PEG-ing out in dementia wards and nursing homes

I t was 1967 when The Beatles released 'When I'm sixty-four' and they – like me – were not yet 30 in a decade when some people encouraged us to trust nobody over that age. In the 1960s, most people in Britain did not live much beyond 75. Far fewer lived for long enough to be at high risk for Alzheimer's and as we shall see in the next chapter if they did get it, they often died rather sooner than they do today. The Beatles were certainly not thinking of a tube–feeding technique called Percutaneous Endoscopic Gastrostomy (PEG), partly because it had not yet been invented. It allows liquidized food to flow straight into the stomach through a small tube that goes through the abdominal wall and keeps many patients with advanced dementia alive.

"Of the many decisions that family members and physicians must make about medical care for patients with dementia", notes a US paper about PEGs, "none is more heart-wrenching than the decision about artificial nutrition and hydration. Despite an extensive bioethical literature arguing that the use of feeding tubes is not mandatory and despite the opinion by a majority of the Supreme Court justices that artificial nutrition and hydration constitute a form of medical care, family members repeatedly state that they cannot let a relative 'starve to death'. [The physicians] often feel they have no choice but to authorize the placement of a feeding tube". However, it wasn't just the family members. "A study of 1446 physicians and nurses found that 34 percent of the respondents who were medical attending physicians and 45 percent of those who were surgical attending physicians believed that even if all forms of life support, including mechanical ventilation and dialysis, are stopped, nutrition and hydration should always be continued."[54]

When I talk to psychiatrists and physicians who deal with elderly patients – and with intensive care physicians who are often asked to resuscitate them – I regularly hear that it is considered 'ageist' to decline resuscitation just because a patient has fairly advanced dementia. They might not resuscitate or actively treat a bed-bound patient who was being tube-fed (though that certainly happens) but they would often resuscitate dementia patients who were still mobile even if they could not recognize family members. Often, this is no longer a matter for clinical discretion; an accusation of ageism will probably lead to internal hospital enquiries and disciplinary procedures, especially if there are allegations that a shortage of beds is a factor in such decisions. Better for your career (and sleep) to cover your back and play it safe. Barely 4% of British patients make written Living Wills but even if they contain 'Do Not Resuscitate' (DNR) requests – which often also specify 'No Tube Feeding' (NTF) – these treatment refusals are sometimes illegally 're-interpreted' unless patients are unconscious or at least so confused or withdrawn that they are no longer able to communicate effectively. That does not describe the many

---

[54] Gillick R. Rethinking the Role of Tube Feeding in Patients with Advanced Dementia NEJM. 2000. 342:206–210

patients with moderately severe dementia or worse who are still able to talk and to respond – if imperfectly and ambiguously – to simple questions. The problem, at least from the point of view of people with dementia whose living wills/advance decisions contain such treatment refusals is that by that stage of the illness, the views they might appear to hold and the answers they might give to doctors and nurses, no longer reflect the views they held when their brains were functioning normally and they wrote their instructions. A treatment refusal that would be valid if a patient were unconscious or unable to respond intelligibly to *any* question about treatment might be overridden, if the patient is nearly but not quite at that stage, by a physician with strong views about 'doing everything', even if the law did not support him. Some patients with dementia continue to request deliverance even when their dementia is quite advanced but others, who had always been in favour of deliverance if they were to get a definite diagnosis of dementia and continued to be in favour when the dementia was still relatively mild, may become ambivalent or lose interest in the idea – and in most other ideas – as the dementia worsens. (See the case of 'Mrs A', discussed in Ch 14.) In any case, many 'no active treatment' decisions are not based on what *patients* wanted to happen when their brains were still functioning well enough to contemplate their management if they became demented. Most of them are written in the case notes as part of a care plan only when dementia is at an advanced stage by *medical staff,* either on their own initiative or after discussion with the family.

According to the consistent findings of the surveys discussed in the next chapter, being kept alive is not what most people in Britain want to happen if they were to develop severe dementia. Many of them, you may not be surprised to discover, are favourably disposed to active euthanasia as well as passive euthanasia – i.e. the deliberate withdrawal or withholding of life-saving treatment with the hope, intention and expectation that the patient will die as a result.[55] Unfortunately, other surveys show that being kept alive is what many of them (and their families) will have to get used to. Despite official recommendations for caution and consultation before inserting PEGs, a 2014 study from Japan – the country with the world-s longest life-expectancy – found 1199 hospital patients and 2160 long-term care home patients aged 65 years or older with PEGs.[56] 62.9% of the hospital patients had "advanced dementia". 61% of the care–home patients had the same diagnosis but whereas only 4.2% of them were said to be "enjoying their own lives" (compared with 16.4% of non–demented patients with PEGs) "approximately 60% of *relatives* [my emphasis] reported satisfaction" with the patients' quality of life.

A 2008 Israeli study of patients in a geriatric centre with various diagnoses found that 36 out of 90 with PEGs had received them not because of *difficulty in swallowing* food but because they were *refusing* food.[57] Their average age was 85.7 years and half of them were still alive a year later. In another fairly recent Japanese study, "more than 20% of patients with dementia lived more than three years after PEG".[58] The fact that guidelines exist which encourage careful thought and consideration of the balance of advantages and disadvantages before inserting a PEG, does not

---

[55] One person who read the MS did not like this term but it seems to be quite widely used and understood.

[56] Nakanishi M, Hattori K. Percutaneous endoscopic gastrostomy (PEG) tubes are placed in elderly adults in Japan with advanced dementia regardless of expectation of improvement in quality of life. J Nutr Health Aging. 2014 May;18(5):503–9. doi: 10.1007/s12603–014–0011–9.

[57] Kimyagarov S, Levenkron S, Shabi A. [Artificial tube feeding of elderly suffering from advanced dementia].[Article in Hebrew] Harefuah. 2008 Jun;147(6):500–3, 575.

[58] Higaki F, Yokota O, Ohishi M. Factors predictive of survival after percutaneous endoscopic gastrostomy in the elderly: is dementia really a risk factor? Am J Gastroenterol. 2008 Apr;103(4):1011–6; doi: 10.1111/j.1572–0241.2007.01719.x.

mean that unwise decisions are now uncommon. One reason may be that financial considerations tend to favour keeping patients alive because dead patients generate no hospital or nursing home fees. The same applies to private hospitals and fee-per-item health services in general. Other reasons, already touched on, are fear of criticism and family pressure. However, in 2004, researchers at a large New York hospital found that many patients with dementia who were admitted for acute medical conditions received PEGs even when the family was not in favour of the idea.[59]

The PEG is a classic example of a simple medical technique, originally introduced for sound reasons, that – partly because of its simplicity – is now widely used for purposes unimagined when it first appeared. A paper describing the history of the PEG notes that while it was developed as a paediatric procedure for infants with anatomical abnormalities or other conditions that made swallowing difficult or impossible, "the latest estimates put the number of PEGs in the United States at 279,000", of which only about 4% had been inserted in children. Many adult patients with gastro-intestinal problems benefit from PEGs and often only need them for a few weeks but it seems that as many as a third of that 279,000 have dementia and the author recognizes that inserting a PEG for feeding problems due to dementia is ethically rather questionable. "Whether or not we should attempt to prolong life is highly controversial. An important final goal should always be to return the patient to oral intake whenever possible, because, among other factors, eating is usually associated with pleasure and provides much needed social interaction. This is particularly true in so many of the tube-fed patients." Unfortunately – at least for the many people who do not want to be kept alive in a severely demented

---

[59] Monteleoni C, Clark E, Using rapid–cycle quality improvement methodology to reduce feeding tubes in patients with advanced dementia: before and after study. BMJ. 2004 Aug 28; 329(7464): 491–494. doi: 10.1136/bmj.329.7464.491

state – patient preferences often come up against "an ongoing need for cost-effective long-term enteral [i.e. stomach or intestinal] access that would permit early hospital discharge of adult patients to nursing facilities. *Indeed, some nursing homes would eventually not accept impaired patients without a PEG."*[60] [my emphasis] Over a period of weeks or months, it is obviously much more cost–effective for a nursing assistant to spend five minutes squirting liquidized food into a PEG than to spend half an hour trying to spoon-feed a confused and reluctant patient, even when the cost of inserting a PEG (which involves intravenous sedation and gastroscopy) is included.

In theory, PEG feeding makes it less likely that frail, enfeebled patients will inhale food and drink into their lungs and develop chest infections. Apart from the fact that many living wills implicitly welcome such infections and other life–threatening illnesses as a way of shortening an undignified, unremembered and unwanted phase of existence, there is not much evidence that PEGs greatly reduce the risk of aspiration, perhaps because some fluid must still be taken by mouth for oral hygiene and comfort. Worse, being tube-fed often means that the patient's hands have to be restrained. Some are simply confused and pick at the tube protruding from the abdominal wall as they pick at the bedclothes, and try to pull it out. Others may retain enough insight and desire for deliverance to pull it out deliberately. To prevent this, the physician "frequently orders the use of restraints. In one study, 71 percent of patients with dementia who had feeding tubes were restrained, regardless of the type of tube used". (It is not only tube-fed patients who are restrained. A resident of Oregon who "used to play football while growing up near Sacramento" but now has Parkinson's

---

[60] Gauderer M. Percutaneous endoscopic gastrostomy and the evolution of contemporary long–term enteral access. Clinical Nutrition (2002) 21(2): 103–110

disease and is campaigning for the 'six-month' restriction of the state's current MAID laws to be removed, complained that: "I'm a big boy.....I see what they're going to do if I get aggressive. They're going to drug me up and tie me down. I've seen that. That's how they treat people that are aggressive in memory care. I don't want to take that chance that I'm going to be there."[61]) That profoundly worrying and depressing description of what amounts to the force–feeding of the living dead was written by Dr Muriel Gillick of the Hebrew Rehabilitation Center for Aged Research in Boston, who is presumably familiar with both religious and non–religious objections to withdrawing food and water. She adds: "There is a pervasive failure — by both physicians and the public — to view advanced dementia as a terminal illness, and there is a strong conviction that technology can be used to delay death. ... Although the use of feeding tubes is not unequivocally futile in all cases, balancing the risks and benefits leads to the conclusion that they are seldom warranted for patients in the final stage of dementia." Dr Seamus O'Mahoney, an Irish gastroenterologist who has written about the excessive and inappropriate use of PEGs told me that their use in dementia was now rare in Britain and Ireland but in a recent paper, he noted that "In our acute general hospitals... [t]he simple, quotidian, social, pleasurable activity of eating has evolved into a medical intervention...that satisfies families, doctors, nurses, speech and language therapists, dietitians, nurses and long-term care homes. Many (possibly most) patients referred for PEG insertion are unable to express their own wishes. PEG may satisfy the complex professional and personal needs of these various groups, but the patient is often the loser."[62]

---

[61] Lehman C. Oregon lawmakers consider expansion of 'death with dignity' law. Jefferson Public Radio in Oregon, 8 March 2019

[62] O'Mahony S. Percutaneous endoscopic gastrostomy (PEG): cui bono? Frontline Gastroenterol 2014;0:1–3. doi:10.1136/flgastro–2014–100521

The English judge who ruled that in severe dementia, tube feeding – with both food and water – could be deliberately withheld in severe Huntington's disease without recourse to the courts, if both the doctors and the family agreed that it should be, may not have realized the implications of his ruling. Advanced dementia of whichever type is still advanced dementia and looks much the same whether it is preceded by the word Alzheimer, Pick, Huntington, Parkinson or vascular. In effect, the judge has ruled that when dementia reaches a certain level of severity, the involuntary (but well-meant) euthanasia of a fellow human being is acceptable, provided it is done slowly and passively by starvation and dehydration, rather than quickly and actively by medication. The inevitable end result of stopping food and water is death from dehydration within a few days. There cannot even be the usual casuistic get-out excuse provided by the doctrine of double effect ('for official purposes, I'm giving this massive dose of morphine to relieve pain and I shall pretend to be unhappy if the patient dies a few hours later') and while the occasional pain-wracked cancer patient rallies for a few days after a good night's morphine-induced sleep that almost but not quite stops their breathing, nobody survives unrelieved dehydration.

The radical – even revolutionary – implications of this development will not be of much interest to people with early dementia who want to die before the dementia becomes more serious. Their intention is to prevent themselves from ever needing to benefit from that ruling. For society as a whole, however, the implications are of great importance, yet the ruling caused little comment, at least in the non-religious media, and that lack of comment seems to confirm those 2007 survey findings which showed that the majority of white British respondents would welcome active as well as passive euthanasia if they became severely demented. For some reason, the media were much more excited when the Supreme Court ruled that the same now applied to patients in a persistent vegetative state. As with the case of Tony Bland (a teenager who was left in a persistent vegetative state after the Hillsborough football crowd disaster) some religious figures and members of disability groups were prominent in their opposition. The illogicality of making a distinction between active and passive euthanasia was something that several of the judges in the Bland case specifically mentioned and were clearly unhappy about. Lord Browne-Wilkinson, one of the High Court judges who made the decision, accepted that "...the conclusion I have reached will appear to some to be almost irrational. How can it be lawful to allow a patient to die slowly, though painlessly, over a period of weeks from lack of food but unlawful to produce his immediate death by a lethal injection, thereby saving his family from yet another ordeal to add to the tragedy that has already struck them? I find it difficult to find a moral answer to that question. But it is undoubtedly the law and nothing I have said casts doubt on the proposition that the doing of a positive act with the intention of ending life is and remains murder."

His fellow appeal judge Lord Mustill wrote: "The acute unease which I feel about adopting this way through the legal and ethical maze is I believe due in an important part to the sensation that however much the terminologies may differ, *the ethical status of the two courses of action is for all relevant purposes indistinguishable. By dismissing this appeal* [against allowing Tony Bland to die] *I fear that your Lordships' House may only emphasise the distortions of a legal structure which is already both morally and intellectually misshapen.*[my italics] Still, the law is there and we must take it as it stands." He also conceded that: "..when the intellectual part of the [appeal process] is complete and the decision-maker has to choose the factors which he will take into account, attach relevant weights to them and then strike a balance, the judge is no better equipped, though no worse, than anyone else. In the end it is a matter of personal choice, dictated by his or her background, upbringing, education, convictions and temperament. Legal expertise gives no special advantage here."

Another important and more recent legal precedent, which has not been appealed,[63] involved Brenda Grant, a woman of 81 with advanced dementia who was tube-fed for 22 months despite a Living Will clearly stating that if she lived to that stage, she should not have any treatment aimed at prolonging her life. The hospital had failed to notice the Living Will and had to pay her family £45,000 in compensation for their carelessness. That case, too, involved the illogical distinction, noted by Lord Browne-Wilkinson, between slow euthanasia by starvation and dehydration and fast or accelerated euthanasia by the administration of sedative drugs over a period that may vary from a few seconds to a few hours or even a few days. You may have more or fewer doubts than the Tony Bland judges that the distinction between active and passive euthanasia is real and not mainly aesthetic but let me present two imaginary – though not wholly unimaginable – cases to show just how illogical and untenable it is.

Suppose you are a physician and have two patients in your care, both of whom have very severe and life-threatening pneumonia. Without intensive care that involves assisted breathing, tracheostomy, intravenous antibiotics, chest physiotherapy and one-to-one nursing, they will almost certainly die. One of the patients is 78 and has dementia that is now at a stage where he sits in a chair for much of the day, increasingly needs spoon-feeding, rarely speaks to anybody and no longer gives intelligible responses to questions. He has led a healthy life and like many Alzheimer patients in their seventies, his heart and lungs have hitherto functioned reasonably well. He has not made a Living Will/advance decision but you know that many Living Wills specifically reject active treatment and resuscitation in this

---

[63] It was an out-of-court settlement.

situation. Were he to recover from the pneumonia, he would probably resume his silent place in the nursing home chair and live for another year or two, though reduced oxygen intake from his infected lungs may have further damaged his brain and accelerated his decline. He has no close relations and you feel that his quality of life is so poor that death would be a kindness; you suspect that like most indigenous British citizens, he would probably not have wanted his pneumonia to be treated in this situation and therefore you do not treat it. You give him small amounts of intravenous fluid – mainly for the sake of appearances and to facilitate the administration of medication – but the only medications he receives are generous doses of sedatives and adequate but definitely non-lethal doses of morphine (because you do not want to be accused of *active* euthanasia) for the painful breathing that is his main and most distressing symptom. After a few somnolent and uncomplaining days, he dies. Most of your colleagues think it was the right decision, though not all of them would have had the confidence to do the same but nobody feels you should face disciplinary action. We shall see in the next chapter that this scenario is often played out in nursing homes.

The other patient is a 28 year old gay man who is HIV positive. He is an international IT consultant and was working and functioning normally before the onset of pneumonia but he gets bad side effects from the anti-HIV drugs that keep most HIV positive patients in good health. Poor compliance with them has left his immune system in bad shape and made him more vulnerable to infections but with appropriate treatment, he will almost certainly return to his premorbid state. However, you happen to be one of those people who strongly disapprove of homosexuality and feel that HIV is God's judgment on him. (His family have similar views and he has no contact with them. As a recent arrival in Britain, he has no close friends here.) You tell your juniors and the nurses to give him a little i/v fluid – for the sake of appearances – but no antibiotics, though in contrast to the older patient's management, you don't feel that his suffering deserves to be alleviated by sedatives, let alone morphine. You are, of course, immediately reported to the management and the police – possibly not even in that order. The patient is quickly transferred to the care of another consultant and he makes a good recovery. You eventually receive both a lengthy prison sentence and a lot of hate mail, as well as some supportive messages from Russia and the Bible Belt.

Below the neck, these patients are clinically almost identical. In both cases, intensive treatment will probably return them to the condition they were in before they got pneumonia. The only difference is that in one case, the quality of the life preserved will be regarded by most people as 'good' while in the other, it will be regarded as 'poor'. Our imaginary consultant is making essentially the same judgment as the judges in the case of Tony Bland, when they chose to regard the poor quality of his life as a reason for ending it without being able to consult him. In most cases, if we want to know the quality of a patient's life, we ask the patient but we already know that the average, not-very-religious British citizen regards severe dementia as synonymous with a very poor quality of life and literally a fate worse than death. Many also regard the quality of the life they would have even with moderate dementia as 'poor'. If they find themselves with early dementia, only a very small proportion actually go to Switzerland or choose self-deliverance but they differ from those who do nothing mainly in their level of determination and their willingness to confront the issue in good time (and also, perhaps, in their financial state). If they were to die during that intermediate stage between early and severe dementia, most would regard the prospect as a fairly unmixed blessing but if pneumonia is, as we shall shortly see, an unreliable (and often unpleasant) escape route from severe dementia, it is even more unreliable in the case of otherwise robust people with less advanced disease.

When there is conflict about the management of an individual patient who lacks capacity, lawyers and doctors are supposed to base their decisions on the patient's 'best interests'. The basic problem is that the default position of the law – like that of many individual clinicians - tends to be that it is always in someone's best interests to be alive rather than dead. In many countries, the law increasingly allows patients to decide for themselves what their best interests are, even if they rate death more highly than life in certain defined situations but doctors do not always accept that principle, even when dementia is not an issue and the patient still has capacity. Not long ago, one British patient had to challenge her doctors in court because they wanted to continue her life-sustaining kidney dialysis against her will. In what became known in the media as the 'champagne suicide' case,[64] a woman in her 60s who had enjoyed, by her own account, a thoroughly hedonistic and even selfish existence involving several marriages, decided that her days of wine and roses were over and asked them to stop the dialysis. Her doctors – including a psychiatrist – thought that only someone who had a serious and sectionable mental illness[65] would make such a request and applied to the court to continue dialysing her under compulsion. The judge not only upheld the patient's view but preferred the opinion of a sensible and experienced solicitor, who thought that she was not mentally ill, over that of the psychiatrist, who thought that she was.

Decisions to withhold treatment in severe but not terminal dementia are even more difficult when patients develop aggressive but not immediately lethal cancers. In contrast to

---

[64] Kings College Hospital NHS Foundation Trust v C and V. Court of Protection [2015] EWCOP 80, Case No: COP 1278226

[65] That is, a mental illness meriting detention under a section of the Mental Health Act

the quick death that followed our imaginary pneumonia, death from untreated cancer would often be both very slow and very uncomfortable. A thought-provoking survey of French patients in the 30 days before their deaths from terminal cancer found that, as might be expected, fewer of the patients who also had dementia received "aggressive treatments"; but only somewhat fewer – 37.7% vs 49.5%. As might also – unfortunately – be expected, patients with dementia were much *more* likely to receive aggressive treatments in private, fee-per-item hospitals. However, that was also true for patients treated in public specialist cancer centres and the differences were large: six times more chemotherapy, seven times more radiotherapy and twice as much artificial nutrition.[66] These findings made the authors ask "an important ethical question". Are these terminally ill patients with both cancer and dementia being *under*-treated or "does the diagnosis of dementia lead to less inappropriate *overtreatment*?" [my italics] They answer: "individuals with cancer [and] dementia might be closer to the adequate level of aggressive cancer care at the end of life than individuals without dementia". Patients with advanced dementia cannot express their own views on the issue but it is clear that many people who make living wills do not want any treatment in this situation, other than good pain relief, and feel that the sooner they die, the better. In France since 2016 (i.e. after this survey was done) all patients who are likely to die within two weeks have the right to receive terminal sedation, which renders them unconscious during that period. However, most patients with advanced dementia will not know or recall that and may not legally be able to request it.

---

[66] Morin L, Beaussant Y, Aubry R, Fastbom J, Johnell K. Aggressiveness of End-of-life Care for Hospitalized Individuals with Cancer with and without Dementia: A Nationwide Matched–Cohort Study in France. J Am Geriatr Soc. 2016 Sep;64(9):1851–7. doi: 10.1111/jgs.14363. Epub 2016 Jul 26.

7

What Do We Want? Euthanasia! When Do We Want It? As Soon As We Need 24-Hr Care!!

Surveys of public and health-professional attitudes to nursing-home care. 'The old man's friend' and treatment decisions in advanced dementia.

When delicate ethical and practical End of Life (EoL) medical decisions are needed, there have been two important changes since 1936 when voluntary euthanasia was debated, in the House of Lords, for the first time in Britain – even, perhaps, in the parliaments of the rest of the world. During the debate, Lord Dawson of Penn, the physician to Buckingham Palace, famously argued that there was no need to legalise voluntary euthanasia (or, by implication, unrequested but patient-friendly euthanasia) because "all good doctors do it anyway". In the 1980s, during the audience discussion that followed a medical debate at which I had spoken, a long-retired surgeon stood up. "When I was a junior surgeon", he said (which must have been around the time of Lord Dawson's one-liner) "if we had any really terminal cancer patients, the consultant would usually say after the ward round 'I think those three should be dead by tomorrow, Perkins, don't you?' and they usually were." Long after he died, Dawson's diaries showed that in that same year, he had personally euthanatized the ailing King-Emperor George V, in the presence of his wife Queen Mary, and his son and heir the Duke of Windsor, with an injection straight into the Imperial jugular vein – conveniently distended from congestive heart failure.[67]

One change is that far fewer people die at home like George V. The other is that treatment is no longer decided (and often administered) by a single physician like Lord Dawson. What a doctor can do in the privacy of the patient's bedroom is very different from what can be done when treatment is planned and administered by a hospital team; when the members of the team rotate every few hours; when new members may come and go from one week to the next; and when medical authority, privilege and discretion – which can certainly be abused but can also be useful – have largely disappeared. Especially when a medical crisis happens at night and requires a major decision, the doctors and nurses on the front line are likely to be relatively junior and lacking the confidence that comes with experience. Today, while littering the field with ever more legal, administrative and professional obstacles and penalties, society still expects doctors to make these difficult decisions routinely. That has not been a justifiable expectation for several decades.

In Britain, what used to be a widespread acceptance of direct family responsibility for continuing care in old age, including elderly members with dementia, has largely died out, along with the extended family households that helped to make it possible. Both the acceptance and the household structures may persist, for the moment, among some ethnic minority communities but a Hong Kong study found that

---

[67] The diaries also indicate that at Queen Mary's request, the timing of the injection was dictated by her desire to release the news of the King's death too late for it to get into the *lumpen* evening press but just in time to make the front page of *The Times*.

"because of changing values…the significance of filial piety is on the decline".[68] In India too, the high level of domestic care for his grandfather described by the surgeon-writer Atul Gawande[69] can no longer be taken for granted, even in families that can afford it. "The large extended family, one of the pillars of Indian society, in which the young care for the old and it is second nature to integrate them in their lives, is disintegrating".[70] Until not very long ago, if a member of a British household with advanced dementia developed life-threatening lung or heart problems, hospital admission was often neither expected nor wanted by the family. GPs could take the whole situation into consideration, including the attitude of the family. They would often consider prescribing an antibiotic, for example, but would not necessarily get the district nurse to inject it if the patient's overall status made swallowing difficult, and feeding-tubes would never be used, though ordinary naso-gastric tubes had been around for a long time. If they knew the family well, as they generally did, they would not usually 'strive, officiously to keep alive' patients with advanced dementia if the family thought that to do so would be unkind. Such patients were generally sent to hospital only if they had little family support or had symptoms that were particularly distressing either to them or to their carers. Both families and nursing homes often accepted that there was 'a time to die' and that interfering with nature's timetable was not always wise or appropriate. If the patient recovered from the pneumonia, well, they recovered. If not,

[68] Mok E, Lai C, Wong F, Wan P. Living with early–stage dementia: the perspective of older Chinese people. J Adv Nurs 2007, 59(6), 591–600

[69] Gawande A. Being Mortal: illness, medicine and what matters in the end. London, Profile/Wellcome. 2014, 14–16.

[70] Merten M. The forgotten ones: the misery for millions growing old in India. BMJ 2018;360:k1040

pneumonia was widely perceived by both doctors and families as not a bad way to go if generous sedation and pain relief were provided. In 2017, the journalist and former Conservative MP Matthew Parris recalled that a "kindly but candid senior nurse, surveying the pitiful ranks of helpless, hopeless, senile old ladies in her care, once put it to me on my Christmas visit...to a rural nursing home in the Peak District: 'In the old days, a good Derbyshire winter would have cut through this lot like a knife through butter'."[71]

I'm not sure that the 'old days' recalled by that candid senior nurse were very far back in time and as we will shortly see, attitudes may not have changed all that much, even if patient management has. The neurosurgeon Henry Marsh, reflecting on the extremely poor prognosis for many patients on whom he had operated for severe brain damage or massive tumours that had destroyed the parts of the brain responsible for awareness and self-awareness, concludes that "the best outcome" would be if they did not survive the operation. Although he felt "unable to let that happen", he continued: "I knew of surgeons in the distant past who would have done just that, but we live in a different world now". Yet even in the mid-1960s, I recall similar considerations involving a woman of 95 with severe dementia who was admitted from her home to the orthopaedic ward on which I was the most junior house-surgeon. She had had an epileptic fit and her bones were so soft that the convulsion snapped a femur in mid-shaft, leaving us with two choices. We could operate and hold the ends together with a metal plate or we could keep her in bed and hold her leg in traction with weights, pulleys and adhesive plaster for twelve weeks. Given her extremely frail state, the very likely (but not absolutely certain) outcomes were a relatively quick death from surgery

---

[71] https://www.spectator.co.uk/2017/05/a-dementia-tax-would-eventually-become-a-euthanasia-bonus/

or a protracted one from bedsores and pneumonia. Both were probably quite painful ways to die and either way, her quality and appreciation of life would be minimal. The consultant opted for surgery. He was not the sort of man to discuss ethical problems but we suspected that he thought it would be the quickest way to end her almost vegetative existence, which it did after three days. We junior medics and the nurses tried discreetly but unsuccessfully to put an end to her suffering before she was submitted to this pointless ordeal. If she had not been demented, we would have tried very hard to keep her alive and we would have felt sad if we had failed but in this case, nobody – including her family – felt strongly that it would have been preferable for her to survive. However, the main point of this story is that all the nurses – including the ward sister – and all the junior doctors thought that we were making the right decision. We were prepared to take the modest risk of acting on it because although not universal, it was a widely accepted practice.

It was even, apparently, accepted by the Director of Public Prosecutions when I wrote an account of it a decade or so later. Someone then publicly demanded that the DPP prosecute me for admitting to attempted murder and I was interviewed by a very amiable detective sergeant at Scotland Yard. When, after a suitable interval, he summoned me back to say that no action would be taken, he added that if he were in that situation himself, he hoped he would be treated by a doctor like me. Many other doctors, before and since that time, have published similar stories, nearly always with a similar lack of prosecutorial response. The official excuse in my case was 'lack of evidence' but I know for certain that the DPP never tried to obtain any evidence in the first place. In an age of social media that has also seen the death of deference, doctors may be less confident of the outcome than I was (as were my professional insurers, the Medical Defence Union, who argued that it was no more than a conventional exercise of clinical discretion) but as we shall see, many clinical decisions identical in their benevolently paternalistic intention to ours are still being made every day. They just involve much more hypocrisy, dishonesty, casuistry and hand-wringing.

By the 1980s, patients' rights and autonomy were increasingly recognized and benevolent paternalism became correspondingly less popular with doctors but it was still very widely appreciated and desired by patients in some situations. I know that because early in that decade, I briefly had a part-time NHS job that involved seeing lots of patients for very short consultations. Often I saw six or eight every hour and it occurred to me that I could easily carry out some simple and informal patient surveys to satisfy my curiosity and provide useful material for the fortnightly column in *General Practitioner* that I wrote for nearly 20 years. One of those surveys asked about the sort of treatment they would want if they ever became demented enough to need institutional care.[72] Nobody asked: 'What is dementia?' and although the qualifier 'Alzheimer's' was not so familiar then, everybody knew that dementia implied the progressive and permanent loss of memory and relationships and the gradual destruction of the personality. In the 1980s, institutional care mainly took place in the large mental hospitals that still existed. Most of them had dementia wards where people with advanced – though not necessarily terminal – dementia were cared for (at the State's expense) until they died. Several of my interviewees had personal experience of dementia in their families.

'If you were ever admitted to such a ward', I asked, 'I'm interested in how you would want to be treated. There are three options.' The first was: 'I would like Matron to put something

---

[72] Another revealed that patients preferred their doctors not to dress very informally.

into my tea to end my life as soon as possible.' The second was: 'The Matron option is a bit too radical but at the first sign of pneumonia or other life-threatening illness, I very definitely don't want to be treated and hope I will be heavily sedated to help me to die.' Option three was: 'I would like to be treated just like any other patient and be resuscitated if I have a serious illness.' None chose option three. They were about equally divided between options one and two.

Several post–2000 papers show that the results of my small informal survey in the early 1980s were very similar to those of larger and more sophisticated studies today. One, involving 725 members of the general public in South-East England,[73] concluded: "In the face of severe dementia, less than 40% of respondents would wish to be resuscitated after a heart attack, nearly three-quarters wanted to be allowed to die passively and almost 60% agreed with physician-assisted suicide. ... Our survey suggests that *a large proportion of the UK general public do not wish for life-sustaining treatments if they were to become demented and the majority agreed with various forms of euthanasia.*" [my italics] That as many as 40% *would* want to be resuscitated may reflect the intriguing additional finding that: "White respondents were significantly more likely to refuse life-sustaining treatment and to agree to euthanasia compared with Black and Asian respondents". I'll return to that last point in Chapter 8.

A recent Dutch survey describes the responses of three groups to two hypothetical end-of-life scenarios. One involved cancer, the other dementia but in both cases, the patients have reached the stage where rational communication is no longer possible. In the dementia scenario, "you...no longer recognise your family or friends. You refuse to eat and drink

---

[73] Williams N, Dunford C, Knowles A, Warner J. Public attitudes to life–sustaining treatments and euthanasia in dementia. Int J Geriat Psychiat 2007 Dec;22(12):1229–34.

and you retreat more and more into yourself. To communicate with you about medical treatments is not possible any more".[74] Respondents were asked to state their preferences in this situation about artificial feeding and hydration, antibiotics in the event of pneumonia, resuscitation in the event of cardiac arrest and artificial respiration. The preferences of 5661 respondents who were members of the Dutch equivalent of My Death, My Decision or Dignity in Dying and had completed living wills, were very similar to those of a representative sample of 1402 Dutch citizens who were not members and had not completed a living will. In both of those groups, a large majority "want to forgo all four [resuscitation procedures]" in both cancer and dementia. A study that compared British and US attitudes to EoL decisions as Mental Capacity gradually disappeared found "a high prevalence of preference for 'measures to end my life peacefully' when decision-making capacity was compromised, which increased as dementia progressed". However, although having previous exposure to dementia increased that preference; "living with children…and being of 'black' race/ethnicity" reduced it.[75]

A survey of elderly people in the Netherlands found that a preference for avoiding life-prolonging treatment in advanced disease with a poor prognosis "ranged from 61% to 79% in cancer and 75% to 88% in dementia scenarios". The authors concluded that "The more frequent desire to forgo treatments

[74] Van Wijmen M, Pasman H, Widdershoven G, Onwuteaka– Philipsen B. Continuing or forgoing treatment at the end of life? Preferences of the general public and people with an advance directive. J.Med.Ethics. Published online September 2nd 2014. 10.1136/medethics–2013–101544

[75] Clarke G, Fistein E, Holland A, Barclay M, Theimann P, Barclay S. Preferences for care towards the end of life when decision–making capacity may be impaired: A large scale cross–sectional survey of public attitudes in Great Britain and the United States. PLoS One. 2017 Apr 5;12(4):e0172104. doi: 10.1371/journal.pone. 0172104. eCollection 2017.

in case of dementia than cancer suggests that *physical deterioration is more acceptable than cognitive decline*".[76] [my italics] Yet doctors – even though they increasingly repeat mantras about patient autonomy and choice – may ignore reasonable assumptions about their patients' wishes and choices when dementia is involved. In a 2002 survey with particularly puzzling and troubling findings, over 500 Finnish doctors were asked how they would deal with two clinical scenarios involving *terminally ill patients* who developed a life–threatening additional illness, one group suffering from cancer, the other from advanced dementia. 83% said that they would not resuscitate the cancer patient but *only 57% of them would not resuscitate in the case of dementia*.[77] Fortunately, Finnish doctors seem to have become less interventionist since that study – but only somewhat less.[78]

The comparatively recent arrival of social media networks has made it easier to do research into public attitudes to MAID in dementia. A team from Auckland University in New Zealand have recently used the opportunity provided by 'netnography' ("a specialized form of ethnography adapted to the unique computer-mediated contingencies of today's social worlds") to

---

[76] Evans N, Pasman HR, Deeg D, Onwuteaka–Philipsen B; EURO IMPACT.
Collaborators (17) How do general end-of-life treatment goals and values relate to specific treatment preferences? a population–based study. Palliat Med. 2014 Dec;28(10):1206–12. doi: 10.1177/0269216314540017. Epub 2014 Jun 18.

[77] Hinkka H, Kosunen E, Lammi EK, Metsänoja R, Puustelli A, Kellokumpu–Lehtinen P. Decision making in terminal care: a survey of Finnish doctors' treatment decisions in end-of-life scenarios involving a terminal cancer and a terminal dementia patient. . 2002 May;16(3):195–204.

[78] Piili RP, Metsänoja R, Hinkka H, Kellokumpu–Lehtinen P,6, Lehto J. Changes in attitudes towards hastened death among Finnish physicians over the past sixteen years. BMC Med Ethics. 2018 May 30;19(1):40. doi: 10.1186/s12910–018–0290–5.

obtain the views of "five Facebook communities (UK, Australia, Canada, US & NZ)" whose followers varied in number from 3,247 to 322,961 and "posted news daily, mainly related to [MAID] in contexts: such as court cases, family assisted deaths, law changes, etc.". There were 1,007 comments on MAID and dementia in response to 316 posts. Noting an apparent "increase in public awareness and concerns/fears in relation to a dementia diagnosis", they conclude that "There is a profound fear of developing dementia and its ensuing physical and cognitive decline, which has made our online members (as public representative) consider alternative end-of-life options such as expressing their preferences in an advance directive, and considering an assisted death".[79]

These surveys strongly suggest that when it comes to actual treatment and despite all the proclamations about equality, non–discrimination and so forth, most people, most potential sufferers, most carers, most doctors and most nurses do not, in practice, regard people with severe dementia, or other adults who develop severe cognitive impairments relatively late in life, in the same way that they regard people of the same age who are not demented. (Attitudes to the severely brain–damaged at the other end of life, touched on in Ch 15, involve additional and very different medical and ethical issues, mainly because children and infants are, almost by definition, incapable – and never have been capable – of understanding these issues and of asking themselves and others the relevant questions.) We may all agree with the principle that seriously ill people without dementia are entitled to the best intensive care that the country can provide (if they want it) and we are pleased if the treatment is successful. We do not all agree – and most of us definitely

---

[79] Views on assisted dying for individuals with dementia: a Netnographic approach. Dehkhoda A, Malpas P, Owens R G. Paper presented at ICEL3 conference Ghent, March 7-9, 2019.

disagree – that the same principles apply to those who also have severe or even moderately severe dementia, including ourselves should we become demented. There is clearly a spectrum of views but many good doctors do not believe that everything possible should be done to treat or resuscitate the severely demented (or people with other severe forms of permanent brain damage, such as persistent vegetative states) and many say privately that they think it is both pointless and a misuse of resources that are not – and cannot be – infinite. However, like the rest of society, many of them are reluctant to spell this out in public, possibly fearing that if they both express their views and act on them, they risk being sued or sanctioned. Those who are reluctant to spell their views out even in an anonymous survey can simply refuse to return the survey – as most Quebec doctors evidently did in a survey discussed later.

Some, like Henry Marsh, are less coy. "It is estimated", he writes, "that there are 7,000 people in the UK in a 'persistent vegetative or minimally conscious state'. They are hidden from view in long-term institutions or cared for at home, twenty–four hours a day, by their families. There is a great underworld of suffering from which most of us turn our faces. It is so much easier to operate on every patient and not think about the possible consequences. Does one good result justify all the suffering caused by many bad results? And who am I to decide the difference between a good result and a bad result? We are told that we must not act like gods, but sometimes we must, if we believe that the doctor's role is to reduce suffering and not just to save life at any cost." Yet if a 'good' outcome in this neurosurgical context means that the patient is able to preserve or regain most of his or her personality, intellect and ability to communicate with others, and if a 'bad' outcome means that these *desiderata* are not achieved, then *all* treatment outcomes in severe dementia are 'bad' because none of the *desiderata* was present to begin with and unlike the occasional neurosurgical success to set against the many vegetative failures, there is absolutely no prospect that a patient with severe Alzheimer will improve, let alone recover.

Younger people also appear to dread the prospect of getting severe cognitive impairments and most would rather be dead than run that risk. When the general public are given honest – rather than over-optimistic – information about the risks of poor quality survival after serious head injuries, they are reluctant to agree to cranial decompression surgery to relieve pressure on the swollen brain that might keep them alive but leave them with the sort of catastrophic brain damage that so worried Henry Marsh. "*If very severe impairment was anticipated, only 1%… favored surgery.*[my italics] With severe, moderate, and slight impairment, the [proportions] were..6%, 24%, and 63%. *The majority of persons does not favor intervention even if only moderate impairment is anticipated*".[80] [my italics]. When a more informed and medically sophisticated group – anaesthetists – were given similar information, "preferences to consent to the procedure changed [significantly] after being informed of the predicted risks of unfavourable outcomes".[81] It is not only doctors who would, as it were, rather be dead than tube–fed.

Pneumonia has often been called, without irony, 'the old man's friend' but it has never been a very reliable friend. A former president of the old Voluntary Euthanasia Society – a minister in the Wilson governments of the 1960s and a Labour peer – suffered a devastating stroke that left him almost unable to speak or read, though he could indicate yes or no to

---

[80] Klein A, Kuehner C, Schwarz S. Attitudes in the General Population Towards Hemi–Craniectomy for Middle Cerebral Artery Infarction. A Population–Based Survey. Neurocrit Care. 2012 Feb 7

[81] Honeybul S, O'Hanlon S, Ho KM, Gillett G. The influence of objective prognostic information on the likelihood of informed consent for decompressive craniectomy: a study of Australian anaesthetists. Anaesth Intensive Care. 2011 Jul;39(4):659–65.

questions. He had made it very clear – both before and after the stroke – that he did not want to be kept alive in such a state and his doctors knew and respected his views. Twice he got pneumonia and twice the doctors did not treat it but he recovered each time. Only with the third attack, several years after he was admitted to the nursing home, did pneumonia release him from the torment which, despite his limited speech, he made very clear to all his visitors.[82]

A 2006 US study looked at 154 patients with *advanced* dementia who "experienced 229 suspected pneumonia episodes during the last 6 months of life". Over half of the episodes were in the final month, which implies that many of the patients recovered from pneumonia before dying from another episode, or from something else. Over 90% received active rather than palliative treatment. "Antibiotic treatment for the 229 episodes was as follows: none, 9%; oral only, 37%; intramuscular, 25%; and intravenous, 29%". In other words, over half were given intensive antibiotic treatment, often involving painful intramuscular injections and the side-effects, such as diarrhoea, nausea and rashes, that are common when antibiotics are given in large doses to frail, elderly patients. Again, it was noted that "the aggressiveness of treatment" is most importantly determined by "advance care planning [and] the patient's cultural background".[83] The problem is that this 'planning' often does not occur until the patient is nearly dead anyway and the 'plan' is often made by the medical and nursing staff rather

---

[82] As a child in the pre–antibiotic age, my father's life was despaired of during the Spanish Flu epidemic of 1918–19 that killed more healthy young men than World War I but he recovered from pneumonia without lasting damage.

[83] Chen JH, Lamberg JL, Chen YC, Kiely DK, Page JH, Person CJ, Mitchell SL. Occurrence and treatment of suspected pneumonia in long–term care residents dying with advanced dementia. J Am Geriatr Soc. 2006 Feb;54(2):290–5.

than by (or in consultation with) the family – if any. "For most institutionalized persons with advanced dementia, a decision to forgo hospitalization" – where aggressive treatment tends to be routine – "is not made until death is imminent. Thus, hospital transfers are common near the end of life". Only a third had 'Do Not Hospitalise' (DNH) orders six months before they died and this had only risen to half in the last month of life [84]

As with advanced cancer, doctors often over-estimate the likely survival time in severe dementia, failing to accept that it is, in its own way, a terminal illness. "At nursing home admission, only 1.1% of residents with advanced dementia were perceived to have a life expectancy of less than 6 months; however, *71.0% died within that period.*" [my italics] Half had a DNR order but only 1.4% had a DNH order. "Non–palliative [i.e. active treatment] interventions were common among residents dying with advanced dementia: tube feeding, 25.0%; laboratory tests, 49.2%; restraints, 11.2%; and intravenous therapy, 10.1%. Residents with dementia were *less* likely than those with cancer to have directives limiting care but were *more likely to experience burdensome interventions*".[my italics] Common and distressing conditions in advanced dementia included "pressure ulcers [i.e. bedsores]…constipation… pain… and shortness of breath". This study is not very recent but not very old either. The ambivalence, confusion and indecisiveness – both ethical and therapeutic – and the high levels of both avoidable and unavoidable discomfort that it reveals are evidently still very common; perhaps 'normal' or 'predictable' would be more accurate descriptions.[85] 'Terminal' has two meanings in this context. It can mean: 'we think

[84] Lamberg JL, Person CJ, Kiely DK, Mitchell SL. Decisions to hospitalize nursing home residents dying with advanced dementia. J Am Geriatr Soc. 2005 Aug;53(8):1396–401.

[85] Mitchell SL, Kiely DK, Hamel MB. Dying with advanced dementia in the nursing home. Arch Intern Med. 2004 Feb 9;164(3):321–6.

death is likely in a few days or weeks' but it can also mean: 'this patient's dementia is now very severe. Conversation is impossible and nothing seems to give her pleasure. She may live for another six months or a year but she will get steadily worse, whatever we do'. A very recent review criticized the frequency with which "incurably dying patients receive antibiotics in their last days or weeks of life, even in patients with 'do not resuscitate' (DNR) or 'comfort measures only' orders.[86] So common have pointless, painful interventions and investigations become in all sorts of manifestly terminal illnesses that the term 'non-beneficial treatment' (NBT) has been coined to describe them. One recent definition is. "Any treatments, procedures or tests administered to [elderly] patients who are naturally dying and which will not make a difference to their survival, will probably impair their remaining quality of life and can substantially cause them pain or prolonged suffering, or leave them in a worse state of health than they were before admission". Unfortunately – and especially when fee-per-item medical systems combine with misplaced therapeutic enthusiasm, inexperience and fear of criticism for *not* 'doing something' – NBTs are common. A 2016 review[87] found that "Evidence from 38 studies indicates that on average 33-38% of patients near the [end of life] received NBTs." In some of the reviewed studies and for some NBTs, the incidence was as much as 90%. It is not easy to change the medical, nursing and administrative cultures that lead to so much pointless, unpleasant and often expensive intervention in what are clearly,

---

[86] Macedo F, Nunes C, Ladeira K, et al. Antimicrobial therapy in palliative care: an overview.   Support Care Cancer, 2018 doi.org/10.1007/s00520–018–4090–8

[87] Cardona-Morrell M, Kim J, Turner RM, et al, Non-beneficial treatments in hospital at the end of life: a systematic review on extent of the problem. Int J Qual Health Care. 2016 Sep;28(4):456-69. doi: 10.1093/intqhc/mzw060.

in most cases, the patients' final days or hours. The 1995 'SUPPORT' controlled trial was a well–planned and energetic attempt over four years to "improve end-of-life decision making and reduce the frequency of a mechanically supported, painful, and prolonged process of dying".[88] It featured "multiple contacts with the patient, family, physician, and hospital staff to elicit preferences, improve understanding of outcomes, encourage attention to pain control, and facilitate advance care planning and patient–physician communication". Before this educational exercise, "38% of patients who died spent at least 10 days in an intensive care unit (ICU); and for 50% of conscious patients who died in the hospital, family members reported moderate to severe pain at least half the time." Even more worrying, nearly half of the Do Not Resuscitate orders were not written until two days, at most, before death. Yet while the pre–educational period of SUPPORT "confirmed substantial shortcomings in care for seriously ill hospitalized adults", the educational intervention "failed to improve care or patient outcomes". The situation in the Netherlands is – depending on your point of view – somewhat better. In one Dutch survey, living wills were surprisingly rare (4.9%) but "in almost half of the residents…decisions were made not to start potentially life-prolonging treatment such as hospital transfer and artificial nutrition and hydration. In…53.7%, decisions were made to withdraw potentially life–prolonging treatment such as artificial nutrition and hydration and medication".[89]

---

[88] (SUPPORT). The SUPPORT Principal Investigators. [No authors listed] A controlled trial to improve care for seriously ill hospitalized patients. The study to understand prognoses and preferences for outcomes and risks of treatments. JAMA. 1995 Nov 22–29;274(20):1591–8.

[89] Hendriks SA, Smalbrugge M, Deliens I. et al. End-of-life treatment decisions in nursing home residents dying with dementia in the Netherlands. Int J Geriatr Psychiatry. 2017 Dec;32(12):e43–e49. doi: 10.1002/gps.4650. Epub 2016 Dec 29.

Nevertheless, a quarter received antibiotics in the last week, mainly for pneumonia. Even if the main purpose of prescribing antibiotics is to reduce the severe discomforts that pneumonia can cause (shortness of breath, painful and rapid breathing, and high fever, often leading to hallucinations or increased confusion) rather than to prolong life, they don't seem to have much effect in frail patients whose respiratory muscles are as weak as their other muscles and who therefore have difficulty in clearing their lungs by coughing or cooperating with chest physiotherapy. "Nursing home residents with dementia and pneumonia experience severe discomfort which increases in the six days preceding death. Discomfort occurs regardless of treatment with antibiotics or not Residents dying from pneumonia experienced more discomfort than residents dying of other causes. Moreover, death from respiratory infections has been associated with the largest symptom burden before death. For example, 78% experienced respiratory distress compared to 40% for residents dying from a cardiovascular disorder". Furthermore, "Because residents with dementia are often unable to express their complaints and wishes about treatment, relieving the symptoms of pneumonia in these residents is particularly challenging". [90] Not surprisingly, "Discomfort and symptoms were higher for residents who died within 20 days from the diagnosis of pneumonia and lower for residents who were observed asleep", which implies that patients who died from pneumonia often failed to get any sleep during their last miserable days and hours on earth. With a 'friend' like that, an enemy might be more attractive.

In moderate and advanced dementia, fractures of the hip are common and often prove terminal, as with my patient with a

---

[90] van der Maaden T, de Vet H, Wilco P. Achterberg W, et al. Improving comfort in people with dementia and pneumonia: a cluster randomized trial BMC Med. 2016; 14: 116. Published online 2016 Aug 11. doi: 10.1186/s12916–016–0663

fractured femur described earlier. The authors of a New York study start from the position that "if their prognosis is poor, then emphasis should be placed on palliative care for these patients rather than on curative interventions". Those same principles and considerations motivated our attempt to save my patient from further and pointless pain. Mortality for patients with advanced dementia six months after a hip fracture was 55%, compared with 12% for age-matched but cognitively intact patients,[91] yet they received "as many burdensome procedures as cognitively intact patients". Worse still, "only 24% of patients with end-stage dementia and hip fracture received a standing order for analgesics".

Without being dishonest or dismissive about the realities of the condition, it is not obvious to me how doctors, nurses or counsellors might effectively dissuade people with early dementia who, having seen the future, want very much to avoid being there when it happens. If they make a living will, it will very probably stipulate palliative care rather than active treatment once dementia is well-established but their ultimate preference would probably be for death to be brought forward as much and as quickly as the law allows – including both passive euthanasia and various shades of the active version. Some patients with early dementia (and their doctors) may hope for breakthroughs in treatment but one can hardly criticise those who don't want to take the risk that any breakthrough may not come in time to save them. It is also vanishingly unlikely that any treatment could restore a severe loss of brain cells and functions, as opposed to halting or preventing the disease process. In any case, Alzheimer experts give us very few grounds for optimism. "Relatively few clinical trials are undertaken for [Alzheimer] therapeutics, considering the magnitude of the problem. The success rate for

---

[91] Morrison RS, Siu AL. Survival in end–stage dementia following acute illness. JAMA. 2000 Jul 5;284(1):47–52.

advancing from one phase [of development] to another is low, and the number of compounds progressing to regulatory review [i.e. near to being licensed] is among the lowest found in any therapeutic area".[92] What Shakespeare called the 'seventh age of man' ('a second childishness and mere oblivion, sans teeth, sans eyes, sans taste, sans everything.') is what some physicians call the 'infantile triad', consisting of incontinence of bowel and bladder, inability to communicate and having to be spoon-fed. It is not most people's idea of a happy ending and the only advance since Shakespeare's time is that these days, many of us – even in our 90s – will still have most of our own teeth.

In Chapter 8, I discuss the largely religious arguments against choosing how and when to die and the interesting ethnic, religious and cultural factors that consistently differentiate the minority of opponents from the large majority in most developed countries who support deliverance and 'not striving officiously'. Here, I simply note that in countries and communities with relatively relaxed views about religious affiliation or the lack of it (which is to say, most of Western Europe, parts of East Asia and much of the Anglosphere outside the USA) public opinion is not just somewhat but *overwhelmingly* in favour of 'not striving' in conditions where the self-perceived quality of life is very poor and recovery is impossible or very unlikely. Equally significant and important is that pro-choice arguments based on personal preferences are commonly reinforced by a desire not to waste both family and state resources on what is widely seen as pointless and harmful care – both medical and social. As the late Baroness Warnock put it in a recent collection of essays: "I simply do not want to be remembered as someone wholly dependent on others, especially for the most personally private aspects of my life, nor can I tolerate the thought of outstaying my welcome,

---

[92] Cummings JL, Morstorf T, Zhong K.. Alzheimer's disease drug development pipeline: few candidates, frequent failures. . 2014 Jul 3;6(4):37.

an increasing burden on my family, so that no one can be truly sorry when I die and they are free".[93]

To many opponents of legalized deliverance, such sentiments are held to reflect dangerous pressures in society. To most people, I think they will be viewed as altruism. Furthermore, what we spend here on a week's residential or hospital care for one person with advanced dementia would fund a lot of rather useful treatments in countries where, in addition to high infant mortality, many adults die of easily treatable or preventable diseases long before they get anywhere near our normal retiring age. Among other organisations, *Médecins Sans Frontières* will benefit in my will from the money that I hope will not be spent on caring for my own body if my brain has gone. I find that thought quite comforting. If – despite my best efforts – I ever get to that stage, I would not want to stay alive just because in my second childhood, I may have developed a fondness for tuneless community singing or mindless television-watching that would be completely foreign to my real, adult, intact personality. One childhood is enough for most people and its correct place is at the beginning of life. Furthermore, most childhoods are the start of something promising and joy-bringing for everyone involved. The childhood of dementia is neither. I mentioned earlier the taboo that seems to exist when it comes to depicting the undignified, depressing, terrifying and exhausting aspects of dementia that affect so many patients and their families. I don't mean by this that nothing can – or should – be done or tried to alleviate the manifestations of dementia, particularly in its early-to-moderate stages; or to help families and carers to find the best ways of managing their personal or therapeutic interactions with the changed and

---

[93] Warnock M, Easeful death for the very elderly. *In*: C. Brewer and M. Irwin (Eds) I'll See Myself Out, Thank You. The arguments for rational suicide. Newbold on Stour, Warwickshire. Skyscraper. 2015. 131–44

changing person who may now be living with them. However, when families are desperate, there is no shortage of people offering to help them. Some are motivated mainly by altruism, others by the (perfectly legitimate) business opportunities that providing such services can offer. Unfortunately, both altruists and businesspeople sometimes suffer from a conviction that they have developed unique and effective interventions that will bring major benefits to patients. Doctors are not immune to such delusions of effectiveness but during the past century of increasingly scientific, evidence-based medicine and surgery, we have learned the painful but necessary lesson that good ideas often turn out not to work; or to have side effects that outweigh the benefits; or that any apparent improvements are due to the arousal of hope and enthusiasm (our own and the patient's) and to placebo and non-specific effects rather than to the specific effects of our new and exciting treatment. For example, the methods developed by the 'Contented Dementia Trust' allegedly make it "possible to *sustain well-being all day, every day, for life,*[my italics] even with a diagnosis of dementia". Some of their advice seems common-sensical ('don't contradict','don't ask questions'; and keep patients occupied). They seem well-intentioned and I got no sense that they are trying to exploit the desperate. Indeed, The Alzheimer Society (see 'List of useful addresses') supports them. They also offer training for carers but when I looked at the 'research' section on their website, I could not find a single reference to the sort of controlled study that is absolutely fundamental to evidence-based treatment. The study that they seemed to rate most highly was an 'evaluation'[94] that did not compare it objectively with any other approach, which makes it rather unlikely that any firm conclusions can be

---

[94] Pritchard EJ, Dewing J. A multi-method evaluation of an independent dementia care service and its approach Aging & Mental Health 2001, 5; 163–72 doi.org/10.1080/13607860020020663

drawn. Given the genuine difficulties of research and treatment in this field, the language of their website is closer to the confident and euphoric claims of 'alternative' medicine than to the more cautious and tentative pronouncements of evidence-based medicine. Their method, it is claimed, "has transformed the lives of the many people we have worked with". Not 'some of' those lives but, by implication, all or most of them. Every face in the leaflet and on the website is smiling, yet most people, it is clear, do not want to live to the stage where nobody ever contradicts them or asks them questions, however kindly their motives. They want to be remembered as the person they always had been; not as the person they have – very unfortunately – become; and certainly not as the person they will finally become, for whom questions and contradictions will be utterly meaningless.

Any research with patients that exposes them to more enthusiastic attention than they would normally have received tends to make both patients and the research team feel better. If the researchers are using a trendy new approach to analysing the results, they will be even keener to believe that their research is an improvement on its predecessors. In this case, they used "Fourth Generation" methodology and valuation, which "identifies stakeholders' concerns, claims and issues about the phenomena being evaluated, then reaches a consensus which is meaningful from these multiple perspectives." Even if any apparent benefits are simply due to increased attention and staff morale, they may not transfer easily to units and institutions staffed by people with less enthusiasm and commitment; or who see working with dementia patients more as a job than as a vocation and do not spend even a moment of their leisure time thinking about how they might do that job better. Working with dementia patients is not many people's first choice. In British nursing homes, carers are often not native English-speakers and may lack the linguistic skills needed to pick up subtle cues, or to respond appropriately when patients refer to local customs and events that are still important to them. It reminds me of another well-intentioned study[95] that tried to discover whether intensive social work would reduce the incidence of further deliberate self-poisoning in those who had already taken one overdose. As in the dementia study, many participants said that they had received 'a lot of help' or that they were 'very satisfied with the service' but the intensive social work made absolutely no difference to the rate of future attempts, compared with the control group who received much less attention.

Good care in early-to-moderate Alzheimer-type dementia will not prevent it from progressing to the late and truly terminal stages. It may even prolong them. Although it needs no justification, the importance of sceptical, scientific attitudes to claims of effectiveness is shown by another bit of dementia research that hoped to improve the management of agitation and did have a proper control group. Agitation is increasingly common as dementia advances and medication often makes matters worse. Non-pharmacological methods for controlling it are often promoted and this study compared a well-planned new approach with ordinary care. Unfortunately, despite six training sessions delivered by graduate psychologists to care-home staff directly involved in providing residential dementia care and good attendance at the training sessions, the new intervention did not reduce agitation compared with the old one.[96]

Some fine legal minds have examined the possibility of requiring compliance with a detailed living will/advance

---

[95] Gibbons JS, Butler J, Urwin P, Gibbons JL. Evaluation of a social work service for self-poisoning patients. Br J Psychiatry. 1978 Aug;133:111-8.

[96] Livingston G, Barber J, Marston L. et al. Clinical and cost-effectiveness of the Managing Agitation and Raising Quality of Life (MARQUE) intervention for agitation in people with dementia in care homes: a single-blind, cluster-randomised controlled trial. Lancet Psychiatry. 2019 Apr;6(4):293-304. doi: 10.1016/S2215-0366(19)30045-8.

decision that not only forbade tube-feeding or any other kind of nutritional assistance such as spoon–feeding but also requested care staff to refuse ordinary feeding, once a specified level of deterioration is reached, *even if the patient requests food or fluids.* For a very thorough discussion of the issues and difficulties involved, I recommend a recent paper[97] by Norman Cantor, emeritus US professor of law at Rutgers University. He sets out very clearly his concern to be remembered as the person he still is and not as the person he would undoubtedly become if he became more than mildly demented. "I care mightily about posthumous recollections of my personality, and I strive to shape my life trajectory (including a dying process) consistently with my personal vision of dignity." While recognizing that "Some people will confront Alzheimer's with a measure of resignation…or they may be hoping for a miracle cure to surface, or they might value whatever interactions they can salvage with their loved ones. They are entitled to pursue that resolute path.", his own living will includes the following passage. "This wish to hasten my post-competence demise is not based on prospective suffering or distress, but rather on my personal vision of intolerable indignity and degradation associated with cognitive dysfunction….In addition, it is important to me to avoid being an emotional, physical, or financial burden on my family and friends, even if they would willingly assume such burdens". If you have read this far in the book, you may well share his wish. Professor Cantor told me that he recently revised his instructions to carers as follows. "My determination not to prolong my life at the described point of debilitation includes rejection of any and all life-sustaining means. This includes simplistic medical interventions such as antibiotics, blood transfusions, and antiarrhythmics, as well as more complex

[97] Cantor N. On Avoiding Deep Dementia. Hastings Center Rep July–August 2018 15–24

interventions like CPR, mechanical ventilation, dialysis, and artificial nutrition and hydration. Indeed, if my dementia or any other affliction has produced inability or unwillingness to feed myself – for example, because of swallowing difficulties, or other eating disorders, or just indifference to eating – I instruct that my caregivers refrain from hand feeding. If I am indifferent or resistant to hand feeding, I do not want to be cajoled, harassed, or in any way impelled to eat or drink."

Professor Cantor concludes that under US law, it would not be permissible for carers – however sympathetic – to honour a living will's stipulation that they ignore requests for food and fluids when the patient develops severe cognitive impairment but is not facing any immediate medical or surgical emergency; and that they sedate him heavily instead. However, at least in the USA, a document called a 'Dementia Directive' is being increasingly talked about and used. It is a very specific form of living will/advance decision, designed for the truly terminal, Belsen-like patients who are becoming indifferent to food and water but perhaps still appear to request them occasionally. It may be increasingly acceptable for patients to request in advance that at this very late stage of the disease, such intermittent and occasional requests should be ignored and that terminal sedation should be administered instead, even if it is given some other name. To my knowledge, the proposition has never been tested under English or Scottish law but I think the judges might not easily agree, despite their clear willingness to accept withdrawal of food and fluid in patients who need artificial feeding. A doctor who gave at least some sedation and analgesia to a mentally competent patient with early dementia who decided to self-deliver by stopping eating and drinking might not suffer either legal or professional penalties[98] (for a more

---

[98] According to correspondence that I have seen between the General Medical Council and another physician.

detailed discussion of VSED – Voluntary Stopping of Eating and Drinking – see Chapter 18) but equally probably, most doctors would not care to take the risk. Yet the capriciousness of the law as regards feeding emerges if we consider another imaginary but quite easily imaginable case.

This Alzheimer patient has reached the stage at which the cognitively intact, pre-Alzheimer Prof Cantor – and evidently many other people, according to the surveys above – would be very happy if he were to get an acute, life-threatening illness. His living will, like the professor's, specifically refuses any treatment other than comfort medication; and its refusals, in many countries, have to be obeyed. With luck – as his intact self sees it – the condition will quickly cause his death. He will either be too ill to eat and drink, or the condition will quickly overwhelm him despite the intake of some food and fluid.

But what if the patient develops instead not an acute condition with generalized life–threatening effects, like pneumonia, but a less acute local condition that affects only his ability to swallow food? Perhaps a slowly growing tumour of the oesophagus or of an adjacent organ such as the lung? The patient is still hungry and thirsty and repeatedly requests food and drink but he is too confused to realise that he cannot swallow and too forgetful to remember that he was equally unable to eat or drink a few hours earlier. By itself, the tumour will not cause his death for many weeks or months if he is tube-fed. It is clear, despite the patient's limited awareness and vocabulary, that he suffers both hunger and thirst and the inability to swallow fluid will surely carry him off in a week or less, yet the living will expressly forbids any assistance with nutrition and hydration, as it forbids the active treatment of the tumour; and it has to be obeyed. Everyone – including the patient – is very distressed and it is likely that everyone (apart from the patient, who cannot understand what is happening) agrees that in this unusual but not unprecedented situation, the only thing to be done is to take the living will's stipulation of 'comfort medication only' to its logical and maximal conclusion: terminal sedation. The sedatives and analgesics are administered at doses sufficient to keep him continuously asleep but not so large as to cause his breathing to cease quickly, though he would also be a candidate for the discreet, Dawson-style unrequested-but-benevolent euthanasia that, as numerous surveys show, still occurs quite frequently even in countries where it is strictly illegal. This terminal sedation means that he no longer asks for food or water – or anything else – but his last days and hours appear to be free of discomfort and distress and his condition causes minimal aesthetic or emotional distress to add to the grief of his family when they visit. Not only is all this perfectly legal in both the US and Britain but any failure to obey the 'no active treatment' stipulations in the living will could expose the doctors or nurses to criminal proceedings for assault. The law does not allow a doctor to do openly what Professor Cantor would prefer at this stage of his Alzheimer's, namely to sedate him to the point that he cannot experience hunger or thirst, but it allows a doctor to do precisely that if Professor Cantor has the good fortune to suffer one particular type of illness. In the absence of that good fortune, he must await the arrival of another type of illness. Without the uncertain but often fairly rapid effects of the Old Man's Friend or a heart attack, that usually means something much slower to bestow its blessings: a more lethal form of cancer, undialysed renal failure, or the accumulated cognitive and bodily dissolutions and multiple indignities of the truly terminal stages of dementia.

I was worried that dementia care in general and advanced dementia care in particular might have improved since I stopped doing general psychiatry in NHS hospitals in 1987. Could it be that the reality is not as depressing as I have described it? I specifically asked the anonymous, NHS old-age psychiatrist mentioned in the acknowledgement section, who read and commented extensively on the text, about this possibility. He wrote: "My main comment is to reassure you that *at no point did I feel that you were significantly out of touch at all with contemporary dementia care, treatment or ethical issues.*" [italics original]. He added that since he had done some general practice before training as an old age psychiatrist, he was confident that the book also "reflects the clinical situation from a primary care perspective."

NB. Appendix 5 (pages 259 – 262) contains blank Living Will/Advance Decision forms that can be cut out (or copied) and completed. Appendix 4 contains specimen forms suitable for dementia planning.

8

Even Worse Than Murder

Religious and other arguments against suicide, deliverance and withholding or withdrawing treatment.

H ere is the Swedish author and physician Axel Munthe writing of his experiences in Paris hospitals around the beginning of the 20th century. "Was I to turn my face away from those eyes who implored my help, long after the power of speech had gone?...[Death] had his eternal sleeping draught but I had also mine entrusted to me by benevolent Mother Nature. When he was slow in dealing out his remedy, why should not I deal out mine with its merciful power to change anguish into peace, agony into sleep? Was it not my mission to help those to die I could not help to live? The old nun had told me that I was committing a terrible sin, that Almighty God in His inscrutable wisdom had willed it so, that the more suffering He inflicted at the hour of death, the more forgiving would He be on the Day of Judgment. Even sweet Soeur Philomène had looked at me disapprovingly when, alone among my comrades, I had come with my morphia syringe after the old padre had left the bed with his Last Sacrament."[99] Munthe was probably not referring to patients with severe dementia but although he had retired from medicine before antibiotics appeared, one imagines that he would have used them extremely sparingly in the pneumonia scenario. As to the supposed post-mortem benefits of terminal suffering, Munthe's near-contemporary and fellow physician-writer Somerset Maugham wondered "when Christianity will have sufficiently decayed for the fact to be driven out of men's heads that pleasure is not hurtful nor pain beneficial".[100]

The argument put forward by that 'old nun' is still pretty much the official view of the Vatican. "Everyone", states the current Catechism of the Roman Catholic church "is responsible for his [sic] life before God who has given it to him. It is God who remains the sovereign Master of life. We are obliged to accept life gratefully and preserve it for his honour and the salvation of our souls. We are stewards, not owners, of the life God has entrusted to us. It is not ours to dispose of".[101] Yet by the 17th century, Swedish-German philosopher Johan Robeck was arguing that if life is a gift from God, then like any other giver of gifts, God gave up all rights of ownership once it left His hands. Anyone can destroy a gift, Robeck argued:[102] an individual act of suicide may be regrettable or even foolish but it is not the supreme sin that the Vatican still proclaims it to be.

During the debate that led to the decriminalization of suicide in 1961, Lord Justice Denning (later a famous Master of the Rolls) said that "for nearly a thousand years suicide has been regarded as the most heinous of felonies ... [because our religion] decreed that ... to commit suicide was invading the prerogative of the Almighty,

---

[99] Munthe A. The story of San Michele.

[100] Maugham WS. A writer's notebook. . London, Readers Union, 1951

[101] Catechism. Part three. Article 5, item 2280

[102] Lady Churchill famously destroyed Graham Sutherland's retirement portrait of her husband, paid for by his fellow-parliamentarians.

by rushing into His presence uncalled for..." Until 1824, he added, "suicides were buried at a crossroads with a stake through their body and until 1882, a suicide had to be buried by night; and ever since 1882 up to this day, according to the law of the Church of England, a suicide is not entitled to Christian burial." It still is Catholic law but until very recently, both churches got round it by pretending that all suicides are not just mentally ill (which could mean mild anxiety or obsessive-compulsive symptoms as well as mild depression or understandable unhappiness) but so seriously mentally ill that they could not be held responsible for their actions. In a criminal trial, you have to be very mentally ill indeed to get away with that and be found 'not guilty by reason of insanity'. Only in 2016 did the Church of England Synod vote – though not unanimously – for a change in Canon Law to permit an ordinary funeral service and burial even in cases of terminal illness and rational suicide.

It was not always thus. Although most of the opposition to deliverance in Britain (and the USA) comes from Christian organisations and individuals, early Christianity, arising as it did in a Graeco-Roman world where suicide was widely regarded as an honourable choice in certain situations, had no strong views about suicide. Early commentators noted that the several suicides mentioned in the Bible were discussed in neutral or even positive terms and some of the early fathers of the church even regarded the death of Jesus as involving elements of suicide. The poet A. Alvarez also emphasises, in his classic personal and historical study *The Savage God,* that early Christianity did not generally or automatically condemn suicide. The Rev. Prof. Paul Badham, an Anglican theologian, has argued recently and persuasively that deliverance is not incompatible with Christian faith[103] and principles and he has been joined by, among several others, former Archbishop Desmond Tutu. Another senior Anglican recruit is Lord Carey, a former Archbishop of Canterbury from the Evangelical wing of the Church, to the obvious annoyance of his episcopal colleagues who insist on maintaining their mediaeval and completely undemocratic right to occupy 26 seats in the House of Lords. (On retiring, several additional bishops then remain in Parliament as Life Peers.) Furthermore, Lord Carey believes that the right to choose deliverance should cover those, such as the late Tony Nicklinson, with stable disabilities or slowly progressive conditions such as Alzheimer dementia, as well as those expected to die within six months.[104]

That tolerant attitude of early Christians changed when Christianity ceased to be a persecuted cult, or just one cult among many others, and became Rome's state religion. Within a few decades, it set out on the path that eventually made it proportionally the largest and most enduring persecutor and slaughterer of religious and philosophical dissenters in recorded history. St. Augustine was the most prominent of the church leaders who decided that suicide was a worse sin than murder, because suicide not only meant leaving life before God allowed you to do so and without formal confession and absolution but was, in effect, criticising God by not accepting the world that He had made. A suicide would thus be guilty of the sin of

---

[103] Badham P. The Christian Case. *In*: C. Brewer and M. Irwin (Eds) I'll See Myself Out, Thank You. The arguments for rational suicide. Skyscraper. 2015, 135–9

[104] "Dear Colin. Thank you for your thoughtful email. Unhesitatingly I am fully with the argument you advance. [That legislation should include patients with early dementia who retain Mental Capacity.] Whilst I am a supporter of DiD I regard it as a step towards MDMD.... My change of heart was greatly influenced by Tony Nicklinson. With warm regards. George Carey." Personal communication 20th Aug 2018.

despair. In 562 AD, the Council of Braga denied funeral rites to all suicides. Before long, it was ordained that even attempted suicides would be automatically excommunicated.

This, I believe, was very much the view of the late Dame Cicely Saunders. She was rightly praised and honoured for her promotion of hospices and palliative care and nobody who met her, as I did (we got on surprisingly well) can doubt her compassion but she held the fundamentalist – or at any rate, post-Augustinian – Christian view that even though suicide is not now a crime, it is still a sin. I heard her say this at a conference in the late 1980s and she wasn't very keen on living wills either at that time.[105] Given her background – an agnostic who experienced a sudden conversion to Evangelical Protestantism early in life[106] – such views are not surprising. 64% of white 'mainline' US Protestants believe that "a person has a moral right to suicide when [he has an] incurable disease" (as do 62% of white US Catholics) but that falls to 36% for white Evangelical Protestants and 34% for black Protestants.[107] When Islam swept over the Judaeo-Christian world, it absorbed these Augustinian attitudes, along with several others. "The Prophet said, 'He who commits suicide by throttling shall keep on throttling himself in the Hell Fire (forever) and he who commits suicide by stabbing himself shall keep on stabbing himself in the Hell Fire'."[108] British surveys

---

[105] I also pointed out to her that her very sensible and much-quoted advice to give a repeat dose of morphine before rather than after the effect of the previous dose had worn off was not a new idea and had been set out in detail in an 1880 textbook by Munk, misleadingly titled 'Euthanasia'.

[106] Richmond C. Obituary in BMJ https://www.ncbi.nlm.nih.gov/pmc/articles/PMC1179787/

[107] http://www.pewforum.org/2013/11/21/views-on-end-of-life-medical-treatments/

[108] Hadiths. Sahih al–Bukhari, 2:23:446

show that for most religions, even those members who identify themselves as active participants mostly support a change in the law, but there are significant differences along what should now be predictable lines. In a 2013 survey, support was 59% for Anglicans and 44% for Roman Catholics but only 23% for Muslims and 6% for the Pentecostal Christian sects that flourish particularly in Afro–Caribbean communities.[109] Interestingly, MPs who identify as Roman Catholic are much more monolithic in their attitudes than their non-Parliamentary co-religionists. As one researcher reported: "There are no surprises in the behaviour of MPs from Catholic backgrounds – all 24 Labour, Conservative and Lib Dem Catholic MPs present voted against the [1997] motion to bring a bill to allow a terminally ill person to obtain assistance in dying from a doctor. Furthermore, Labour Jim Dobbin and Tory Ann Widdecombe were both tellers for 'No'. On the other hand, there is a split along the party lines among the members from Jewish backgrounds. Five of eight Labour – and the only Liberal Democrat – Jewish MPs present supported the motion compared to the Conservative Jewish Members who unanimously opposed it. The proportion of Labour and Lib Dem Jewish Members who voted to pass the motion is, in fact, higher than that of the rest of the House – 2:1 to 2:3 – that largely voted against the motion."[110]

In contrast, other world religions – Buddhism, Confucianism, Hinduism – either encouraged suicide in some situations (e.g. the ritual of *suttee* for Hindu widows) or at least did not routinely vilify the deceased, refuse conventional funeral rites

---

[109] http://www.religionandsociety.org.uk/uploads/docs/2013_05/1368520681_Summary_Press_Releases_FD2.pdf

[110] Kolpinskaya E. 'Playing roulette with the human life': Religion and parliamentary debate on assisted dying and euthanasia, 1997–2012. Paper presented at 2015 Political Studies Association annual conference (quoted with permission).

for the grieving family or ritually desecrate the corpse. Eastern Orthodox Christianity's position was also very different from Rome's and the Byzantine 6th century Code of Justinian took a sympathetic view of suicides, provided that they were not trying to escape punishment for a crime.[111] Early Christians were willing to criticize the prevailing political power structures but after Augustine, Western Christianity increasingly sided with the rulers of the day. After the Vatican's 7th century anathema on suicide, those Western rulers – adapting Rome's view that people were the property of God and could not remove themselves from life without God's permission – decided that people were the property of Earthly rulers too and treated suicides, unless suffering from obvious insanity, as enemies of the state. Non-insane suicides generally had their property confiscated by the state, the church, or both but many suicides were therefore ruled insane by sympathetic juries to protect them and their families from legalized destitution.

Despite Christianity's historical distaste for suicide, until relatively recently it had much less of a problem with homicide and it wasn't just Catholic Christianity and its Inquisition. In 1553, the celebrated Spanish physician and theologian Miguel Servetus, discoverer of the pulmonary circulation of the blood, was burned alive in Geneva on the orders of John Calvin – along with his books – because of a disagreement about the nature of the Trinity. Just over 300 years ago, a young Edinburgh student, Thomas Aikenhead, was hanged with the full approval and encouragement of the religious leaders of the time for expressing disbelief in God. That was the last such execution in Britain but similar manifestations of Christian morality continued in France until the 1770s and in Spain until 1826 –

---

[111] Code of Justinian Title 50. Concerning the property of those who commit suicide.

the Inquisition's last victim being a mere post-Enlightenment deist. They still happen under Islam. It both amuses and irritates me to be regularly lectured on the sanctity of human life by the spiritual descendants of Calvin and Torquemada.[112] Another ironic feature of religious opposition to deliverance is the way in which religious leaders who officially reject each other's central doctrines band together to obstruct deliverance legislation.[113]

Given this cultural and historical background, it is not surprising that the various types of deliverance arouse feelings that are both strong and often conflicted. Professor June Andrews, a nurse-academic and former director of the Dementia Services Development Centre in Stirling admits that although "I often hear people saying, 'I'd rather kill myself than have dementia…' Suicide is sad and desperate, and it goes against my religious upbringing, even though I'm not very religious now. My horror of it is visceral."[114]

As discussed in Chapter 7, there is majority support for deliverance in terminal illness even among practicing Catholics and – less surprisingly – Anglicans. However, together with conflicted views about deliverance, it seems that the more religious people are, the more they are likely to demand that

---

[112] "..the first official executions of heretics were recorded in 385. They were followed by literally millions of other victims, and during its long reign as an established faith, Christianity claimed more violent deaths than any other religion. Indeed, no system of any kind has equalled the terrible record of persecution inflicted on infidels, pagans, heretics, witches and Jews through inquisitions, ….through propaganda, harassment, imprisonment, torture and death by the Christians over a millennium and a half." Walter N. Blasphemy Ancient and Modern. Rationalist Press Association. London . 1990.

[113] For example, Islam rejects Christianity's central claim that Jesus is the son of God and died on the cross.

[114] http://juneandrews.net/blog/post.php?s=2016–12–26–suicide–and–dementia

'everything possible must be done' even when the unanimous view of the doctors dealing with the case is that further treatment would be futile. That seems paradoxical. After all, if people believe that only God should decide when we die, then surely all life-saving medication and surgery are in some sense interfering with God's plans. (Plans, incidentally, which apparently included the absence of effective interventions for most illnesses until about the last hundred years of the 80-plus millennia of human existence.) Until an eyeblink ago, historically speaking, bacteria and viruses used to kill half of our children before they reached puberty. On this reckoning, cancer, motor neurone disease and Alzheimer's are all, presumably, part of 'God's plans' and we doctors spend our entire professional lives trying to thwart them. It is probably no coincidence that the first person to publish an atheist tract in England and live to tell the tale was a doctor – Matthew Turner of Liverpool – though it was not until 1781 that he felt it was reasonably safe to do so.[115]

As Henry Marsh discovered after assisting a neurosurgical colleague in Nepal, the more ignorant, uneducated, unsophisticated and superstitious the families were – which, I'm afraid, often also meant the more unimaginatively, uncritically and devoutly religious they were – the more unrealistic and insistent were their demands for inappropriate treatments. Notice that I say 'inappropriate' rather than 'useless'. Such treatments can be of no use to the patient but they are very useful to families who refuse to face reality, even when a second or even a third and a fourth honest and independent opinion points to the overwhelming unlikelihood of any return of useful levels of consciousness.

This is an appropriate place to return to the 2007 population

---

[115] In 'Answer to Dr. Priestley's letters to a philosophical unbeliever'. See: Wootton D. New Histories of Atheism In: Hunter M and Wootton D Eds. Atheism from the reformation to the enlightenment. Oxford. Clarendon, 1992

survey in South-East England that showed Black and Asian Minority Ethnic respondents to be much more wedded to the idea of actively treating and, if necessary, resuscitating people with severe dementia who develop a life-threatening illness. I realise that in examining this issue, I may be poking at a nest of particularly hypersensitive and politically–correct hornets but I insist that this marked contrast with the views of indigenous British respondents (and of nurses and carers in Quebec) is related not to their skin colour but to their predominant religions and cultures and that view is strongly supported by the results of the final part of the Dutch survey[116] that was discussed in Ch 7.

As in most countries of North-West Europe, doctrinaire religion is of minor and diminishing interest to the average indigenous Dutch adult but in contrast, the remaining group in that survey consisted of 1059 members of a "Christian-oriented" patient organisation which encourages its members to complete, in contrast to conventional living wills, a "wish-to-live statement". This predictably rejects "actions with the purpose of actively terminating life". It also, in theory, rejects "excessive, medically futile treatments at the end of life" as well. Yet in practice, of this largely White Protestant group that also had fewer years of education than the other two Dutch groups, even when dementia or a terminal illness meant that "personality annihilation" had occurred and meaningful communication was impossible – and almost certainly would never be possible again – 71% definitely or probably wanted artificial feeding and hydration, 67% wanted antibiotics for pneumonia, 59% wanted breathing assistance and 47% wanted resuscitation after cardiac arrest.

---

[116] Van Wijmen M, Pasman H, Widdershoven G, Onwuteaka– Philipsen B. Continuing or forgoing treatment at the end of life? Preferences of the general public and people with an advance directive. J. Med.Ethics. Published online September 2nd 2014. 10.1136/medethics–2013–101544

Unusually for a psychiatrist, I have worked in Intensive Care Units (ICUs) because during part of my clinical career, I detoxified several hundred heroin addicts under general anaesthesia in some of London's best private hospitals. The other patients in the ICUs were mainly post-operative or recovering from severe heart or lung problems but there were usually a few beds around which a group of black-clad women were to be seen at all hours of the day. The patients in those beds had usually suffered massive strokes or head injuries several weeks or months previously and would never recover any ability to communicate. Without intensive care, they would have died rapidly and naturally in the Gulf States where most of them lived but the families of these severely brain–damaged and deeply unconscious patients wanted their other vital organs to be kept going artificially for as long as possible. Most of them needed tracheostomy or mechanically–assisted breathing and all needed to be tube-fed. The Gulf States were apparently willing to pay for this staggeringly expensive exercise in futility and the private hospitals that housed the ICUs were naturally not averse to having a few beds that were regularly and consistently filled with these nice little earners (well over £1000 a day in 2002). Eventually one of the experienced and very highly qualified ICU nurses asked if he could work full–time with my patients – both before they were admitted and during their post–detoxification management – because he was "fed up with keeping dead patients alive". He became one of my most valued and well–liked colleagues and co–authors until his untimely death in an accident. In Belgium, where voluntary euthanasia is legal, recent surveys among its sizeable Muslim communities found that in both first– and second–generation residents "an absolute rejection of every act that deliberately terminates life, based upon the unconditional belief in an afterlife and in God's sovereign power over life and death." was the norm.[117]

Similar cultural differences in attitudes to resuscitation regardless of the likely outcome are found in the US between White and Afro-American respondents and to a smaller extent, between White and Latino respondents. Most members of all three groups are at least nominally Christian but they differ in the level of their attachment to their faith. Both Afro-Americans and Latinos are consistently found to be more religious than White Americans and the same holds true for British residents of African and Afro-Caribbean descent and for the British Muslim population. Paradoxically, when on the brink of death, and even though both religions envisage an enjoyable afterlife (about which Islam gives the most confident, detailed and lyrical descriptions) it seems that the more faithful the adherents, the keener they are to keep their barely–functioning bodies and minds in this imperfect world rather than sampling the joys of the next, compared with those who have less or no faith. Of greater concern they are also less likely than the average secular European resident (of whichever ethnic group) to allow their organs to be harvested after death for life-saving transplant surgery.[118] "Research suggests that individuals who are younger, female, have higher education levels and socioeconomic status, hold fewer religious beliefs, have high knowledge levels, know others with positive attitudes, are more altruistic, and have fewer concerns about manipulation of the body of the deceased donor are more

---

[117] Ahaddour C, Van den Branden S, Broeckaert B. "God is the giver and taker of life": Muslim beliefs and attitudes regarding assisted suicide and euthanasia. AJOB Empir Bioeth. 2018 Jan–Mar;9(1):1–11. doi: 10.1080/23294515.2017.1420708. Epub 2018 Jan 29.

[118] Boulware LE, Ratner LE, Sosa JA, Cooper LA, LaVeist TA, Powe NR. Determinants of willingness to donate living related and cadaveric organs: identifying opportunities for intervention. Transplantation. 2002 May 27;73(10):1683–91.

likely to have positive attitudes toward donation and are more willing to donate their organs."[119]

The deliverance-rejecting, resuscitation-demanding British Asian respondents were probably from South Asian and predominantly Muslim or Hindu backgrounds. Asians from further east have different views, much more like those of indigenous British citizens. In South Korea, where roughly a third of the people are Protestant or Catholic, a sixth are Buddhist and the rest either have no belief or follow traditional Korean versions of shamanism, a 2014 survey by the state–run Institute for Health and Social Affairs showed that "88.9% of 10,452 people aged 65 and over said they object to continuing medical care to prolong life without the possibility of recovery, while [only] 3.9% chose to support continued treatment." Furthermore, "over 80% of 300 elderly people responded in 2015 that they would 'accept death and spend their final days preparing to die a natural death', while the rest said they would fight it with every medical aid available."[120]

It is not only patients and their families whose views on the appropriateness of end-of-life interventions are strongly affected by the religion into which they happened to be born and have important consequences for treatment requests and decisions. Such considerations affect doctors and nurses as well. One recent study that examined the association between attitudes to withdrawing food and water in advanced dementia not only noted significant effects of religious belief and attitudes but also cautioned that "It might be considered more acceptable if physicians and nurses only allow their religious beliefs to influence decision–making if these beliefs are shared by the patient and the relatives, but it could be unethical if this happened

[119] Wakefield CE, Watts KJ, Homewood J, Meiser B, Siminoff LA. Attitudes toward organ donation and donor behavior: a review of the international literature. Prog Transplant. 2010 Dec;20(4):380–91.

[120] Pilot 'right to die' program gets warm reception in South Korea. The Korea Herald/Asia News Network / October 26, 2017

if such beliefs were not shared".[121] As to Intensive Care Units, although it is unlikely that many patients with advanced dementia would be admitted to ICUs, if they do get that far, they (or their families) could find that 25% of ICU physicians "would [not] respect a competent patient's refusal of a potentially life–saving treatment…More Protestant (84%) than Catholic (73%) or Jewish (67%) professionals would follow a competent patient's wish to refuse a treatment that might be lifesaving".[122] The study found that geography (northern vs southern Europe) and "considering [oneself] religious", rather than being just nominally "affiliated" to a given religion, were important predictors. Indeed, in other medical contexts, the north vs south factor can even operate within a country. A BBC report noted that although abortion has been legal in Italy since 1978, "The proportion of Italian gynaecologists refusing to carry out abortions in 2013 was 70%, according to Italian government figures. In southern Italy the proportion was even higher and in Sicily it was 87.6%".

There were too few responses from Muslims for statistical analysis but "Religious nurses and families almost consistently wanted more extensive treatments than those [nominally] affiliated in the same religion if they were terminally ill or permanently unconscious. More religious doctors, families and patients wanted to prolong their lives as long as possible compared to affiliated respondents". The differences can be surprisingly large. A study covering end-of-life decisions in the ICUs of 17 mainly European countries found that "Median time from admission to ICU to first limitation of therapy varied by physician religious affiliation. It ranged from a median of 1.6

---

[121] Rurup M, et al. Attitudes of physicians, nurses and relatives towards end-of-life decisions concerning nursing home patients with dementia. Patient Educ Counsel 61 (2006) 372–380

[122] Bülow H-H, et al. Are religion and religiosity important to end-of-life decisions and patient autonomy in the ICU? The ETHICATT study. Intensive Care Med. 2012. 38:1126–33

days when the physician was Protestant to a median of 7.6 days when the physician was Greek Orthodox".[123] These large and important differences are very relevant to my suggestion in the final chapter that patients and their families ought to be able to choose – directly and/or via living wills – the policies and the religious and philosophical attitudes of the staff of institutions responsible for the care of people with well-established dementia; which means that those policies and attitudes need to be known and publicized. The average sensible citizen would not, after all, choose an avowedly Catholic family planning agency, or a clinic exclusively based on the quasi-Biblical doctrines of Alcoholics Anonymous, for unbiased advice on the full range of contraceptive techniques or addiction treatments.

Not that all Catholic clerics would refuse to provide pastoral care for Catholic patients who decided to seek deliverance, despite their church's official policy of denying them normal funeral rites and burial in consecrated ground. Gabriel Ringlet, an ordained priest who is also the Pro-Rector of the Catholic University of Louvain la Neuve in Belgium even managed to persuade the local Bishop to allow a memorial service, in a Catholic church, for Christian de Duve, a professor of medicine and Nobel Laureate at the same university who had announced his intention, widely reported in the national media, to die by euthanasia instead of waiting for cancer to kill him.[124] The French title of Ringlet's book is taken from St Francis of Assisi: 'You lay me naked on the naked earth'. Its subtitle, 'spiritual accompaniment through to euthanasia', reflects Ringlet's argument that even if one has personal or doctrinal reservations about any form of MAID, religious

---

[123] Sprung CL, et al The importance of religious affiliation and culture on end-of-life decisions in European intensive care units. Intensive Care Med (2007) 33:1732–1739

[124] Ringlet G. Vous me coucherez nu sur la terre nue: l'accompagnement spiritual jusqu'à l'euthanasie. Albin Michel 2018. 77

patients who choose MAID – and their families - still need and deserve spiritual comfort. One hopes that this little local triumph of humanity and compassion over dogma and cruelty is a sign of things to come. Ringlet also describes how an elderly Carmelite nun, driven by the unrelievable pain of her illness to seek euthanasia against her beliefs, sought and received absolution from him. Indeed, just as Dr Johnson famously remarked that 'when a man knows he is to be hanged in a fortnight, it concentrates his mind wonderfully', Ringlet implies that it may be easier to provide good terminal *spiritual* care when both patient and priest know the precise timetable of departure. He stresses the need for appropriate rituals – religious or otherwise – for this "moment of exceptional intensity".[125] Evidently Ringlet is also familiar with the limitations of good palliative care (for many years, Belgium has rated highly in international comparisons) since he describes in distressing detail a woman with a cancer that was slowly eating away her face, making her look increasingly hideous and emitting such an appalling stench from rotting flesh that both her children and her nurses found it difficult to enter her room. In 2000, a British researcher, whose study was based on several months as a hospice volunteer, reported a similar case. "The stench created by Annie – who lingered for six weeks – reached to the reception area and was so dreadful that badly-needed beds vacated by dead patients were not refilled."[126]

---

[125] About 100 miles from Louvain, just over the French border in the tiny village of Étrépigny, the popular local priest Jean Meslier provided the comforting rituals of life and death for his parishioners for forty years, even though a 550-page manuscript found at his death-bed in 1729 revealed that he was an early agrarian socialist who did not believe in any god and disapproved of monarchy. That makes him Europe's first identifiable post-Classical atheist to have put his heretical thoughts down on paper.

[126] Lawton J. The dying process. Patients' experiences of palliative care. Abingdon, Routledge. 2000.

In March 2019, Dignity in Dying (DiD) released a report[127] that showed how faith-based organisations – including some from the USA Religious Right – were prominent among the major funders of opposition to MAID in Britain. Some of the organisations had been equally active in opposing abortion in Britain and the USA. The American ones, in particular, had also been actively encouraging governments in African and other developing countries to impose severe penalties, including execution, for male and female homosexuality, even when it involved behaviour in private. The determination and deviousness of these groups was shown when a BMJ online poll was more or less 'hacked' by opponents, many of whom were very likely to have been religiously motivated. According to Richard Hurley, a deputy editor of the BMJ, "In 2012, 'Should doctors' organisations be neutral on assisted dying?' received 6592 votes" and while multiple voting happened on both sides, "At least one robot was at work…: a single IP address registered in the Westminster area has regularly voted No almost 2000 times…the top 12 IP addresses for multiple votes have cast 4000 votes between them, 3999 for No."[128]

The DiD report did not surprise me because in 2015, I had some correspondence with Living and Dying Well, one of the organisations named by DiD. After meeting one of their officers, I wrote to her:

"Two or three years ago, one of your people spoke at a meeting organised by the Secular Medical Forum. Afterwards, we had some email correspondence but he refused to give me any information about the religious affiliations of any of your board members, claiming that it was irrelevant, because

---

[127] Exposing the anti-choice networks trying to deny doctors a voice. London, Dignity in Dying.

[128] https://blogs.bmj.com/bmj/2018/02/15/richard-hurley-end-of-life-care-the-assisted-dying-debate-continues/

you only dealt in facts. When I tried to look the members up, many of them seemed to be not just religious but actively so. Could you please tell me something about the religious attachments and activities of your current board and of any other major supporters? I'm sure you will agree that these are indeed relevant and also matters of public interest."

She replied "Living and Dying Well does not hold information on what, if any, religious affiliations its board members or others have. Whether individuals have religious beliefs, and if so what those beliefs are, is a matter for them – and for them alone. Our focus is on exploring the evidence surrounding the end-of-life debate, in which a range of views may be taken by people of all religious faiths and none." A further query ("I could not immediately find the names of your board members and major individual patrons or supporters on your website. Could you please let me have them and then I can make my own enquiries.") received no reply.

Living and Dying Well describes itself as providing 'hard evidence and rigorous analysis in place of spin and sensationalism'. Its work is 'supported by experts in the end-of-life debate' but every one of them happens to be strongly opposed to MAID in any form, several of them fervently so and often on apparently religious grounds. One of their patrons is Lord Mackay of Clashfearn, a former Lord-Advocate of Scotland. He was raised in the Free Presbyterian Church of Scotland – a sect so intolerant, extremist and un-ecumenical that it suspended Lord Mackay, even though he was an Elder of the church, for the grave sin of attending a Roman Catholic funeral mass for one of his judicial colleagues. As recently as 2013, it wrote to Prince Charles to complain of his presence at a requiem mass for one of his cousins. Although Lord Mackay's Wikipedia entry describes him as a 'moderate', it adds that "he is a strict sabbatarian, refusing to work or travel on a Sunday, or even to give an interview if there is a chance it could be rebroadcast on the Sabbath".

Among the organisation's new directors appointed in December 2018 was Lord Alton, who (Wikipedia again) "has been appointed to two Roman Catholic orders of chivalry; he is a Knight Commander of Merit of the Sacred Military Constantinian Order of Saint George…and a Knight Commander of the Order of St. Gregory the Great". DiD describes him as "perhaps the most fervent campaigner against abortion rights in the House of Lords". Of equal significance is DiD's discovery that Living and Dying Well has been extensively funded by the Catholic Bishops' Conference of England and Wales and that in 2015, the Catholic Trust for England and Wales provided 'core funding support'. Another new director was Baroness Finlay, a professor of palliative care and very prominent opponent of MAID. In 2012, she received a grant from the Catholic Church of New Zealand when she travelled there and spoke against MAID at a public meeting. She is so fervently and famously opposed to MAID that she has even conjured up a novel objection: that a drug-induced death can be very unpleasant. While – as noted elsewhere – some deaths can be prolonged and distressing for uninformed onlookers, and there was a single case of a patient who took an inadequate dose and woke up, this is actually an argument for more rather than less medical assistance, since deaths are never prolonged when a doctor can be in charge of the whole procedure, as in Canada, Belgium, Holland and Colombia. Baroness Finlay's baseless objection conveniently ignores the numerous reports of deaths which – despite good palliative care – are horrible, painful, exhausting, undignified, malodorous, heart-breaking to watch and truly prolonged.[129]

Some US Evangelical Protestants who are financing

---

[129] Lawton J. The dying process. Patients' experiences of palliative care. Abingdon, Routledge. 2000, passim.

British anti-MAID groups are almost as opposed to Roman Catholicism as they are to MAID. However, many of the groups are anti-abortion largely because they regard women as second-class citizens whose basic job is to produce children at the behest of their masters. They have clear Biblical support for this view.[130]

Let me return briefly to the 'sin of despair' that so worried early Christians and evidently still worries some modern believers. Writing about the depressing growth of conspiracy theories, the journalist Nick Cohen discussed how easy it is to despair and how important it is to resist that temptation. He noted that the exiled Austrian Jewish writer Stefan Zweig committed suicide (together with his wife) in Brazil in February 1942 after making it clear that he feared the triumph of evil, having already left Britain for the USA because he did not feel safe enough. Cohen presumably meant to imply that if only Zweig had hung on until the victories at El Alamein in November of that year and Stalingrad in the following February, he would have stayed alive. "The alternative to despair", according to Cohen, "is to fight and find a pleasure in fighting.[131] That may be true for situations in which the outcome is uncertain. Presumably, even some Jews who were pretty sure of the fate that was planned for them at the end of the railway line to Auschwitz hoped that they might somehow escape it, or would at least go down fighting. Unfortunately, Alzheimer's kills all its prisoners unless they die of something else beforehand. Escape is impossible and fighting needs a sharp brain that can

---

[130] "But I do not allow a woman to teach or exercise authority over a man, but to remain quiet. For it was Adam who was first created, and then Eve. And it was not Adam who was deceived, but the woman being deceived, fell into transgression. But women will be preserved through the bearing of children if they continue in faith and love and sanctity with self-restraint." (New Testament. 1 Timothy. 2:10-15)

[131] Cohen N. Cranks have turned the world upside down – it's time to fight back. The Observer Sat 17 Mar 2018

learn from experience. For those who cling to the hope of a cure, it is difficult to see how even a treatment that effectively prevented Alzheimer's or halted its progress could restore dead brain cells and damaged neural connections.

Not all opposition to deliverance comes from believers. The most prolific non-religious opponent of Medical Assistance in Dying in Britain is Kevin Yuill, a lecturer in history at the University of Sunderland. For the details, I refer you to a scathing review by Ian Brassington of Yuill's main work *Assisted Suicide: The liberal humanist case against legalization*[132] and to the work itself but for a flavour of his arguments, here are a few extracts from that review. "[Yuill writes] 'Legalizing assisted suicide is wrong because suicide should be an individual decision in order to assign responsibility, because it robs the purposeful ending of a life of its dramatic power and shields such an act from judgment.' Whether or not the life in question is bearable is of secondary importance; what really concerns Yuill here and elsewhere is that we should be able to hold the suicide accountable – perhaps to praise, but also to blame and to forgive: 'Suicide involves an individual voluntarily renouncing his own existence but in many cases…renouncing the world. Of course, such an action requires our judgment upon it.' More: allowing doctors to assist will 'remove the moral taint from suicide'. This is simply vile" says Brassington, "and anyway, the claim of the legalisation camp is that there is no moral taint to begin with, and so nothing to remove. A person who wants not to be alive any more, and who seeks help, should not be blamed, and does not need forgiveness; it's a piece of monumental arrogance to think otherwise. Yuill

---

[132] Yuill K. Assisted Suicide: The Liberal, Humanist Case Against Legalization. Basingstoke/ New York: Plagrave Macmillan, 2013

wants us to blame the defeated."[133]

Yuill also supports the principal objections of the disability lobby (discussed in more detail in Chapter 15) because "[s]aying that people who suffer from, say, multiple sclerosis should have the right to legal assisted suicide, [sic] implies that all sufferers of MS [Multiple Sclerosis] live fairly inferior and expendable lives". Brassington disagrees, as I do. "Must we accept this, though?" he asks. "There's no obvious reason to think we should. For sure, it might be that a lot of people think that life with MS is inferior to life without it – given the choice, I wouldn't be indifferent, and I guess a lot of people who have MS would prefer that they didn't as well, which implies that a life with MS is inferior to one without. That, in fact, is exactly why we tend to applaud research into prevention and cure, and why we think that drugs to ameliorate the condition are desirable. In the absence of a cure, it might be that some sufferers do come to believe that the quality of their lives falls so far short of what is tolerable – so inferior to a pre–symptomatic life – that ending them is desirable. Such a belief may be perfectly reasonable: each of us probably has a line below which we would not want to fall. Does it follow from this that we think that MS sufferers' lives, or the sufferers themselves, are expendable? Not a bit of it. Does saying that individuals should be able to seek assistance to die imply that all people in a similar situation are expendable? Of course not." About the only positive thing one can say of Yuill's arguments is that at least they do not invoke the 'slippery slope'.

---

[133] Brassington I. http://blogs.bmj.com/medical–ethics/2013/07/03/book–review–kevin–yuill–assisted–suicide–the–liberal–humanist–case–against–legalization–2/

9
Slippery Slopes: are they always a bad thing?

Opponents of deliverance typically invoke at least two separate slippery slopes. One criticism focuses on the observation that when deliverance is permitted, the number of people who want it increases. Let us immediately remind ourselves, though, that by legal definition and in all the relevant jurisdictions, these people must have the Mental Capacity to make decisions about the current and future management of their conditions. As a rule, their views about deliverance have developed over several years and they are not under any pressure from others to choose deliverance. For most users, deliverance simply means that after much thought, they have exercised their right to choose an alternative end-of-life scenario to the one that is becoming increasingly and unacceptably unpleasant – or looks as if it will do so before much longer. Why is it either surprising or undesirable if it attracts more than a very few followers?

Some critics may not oppose deliverance on principle and might even use it themselves if the need arose (particularly if they are physicians) but often it seems that they do not fully accept the argument from autonomy as it affects the relationship between doctor and patient – an argument that accepts the basic, presumptive right of adults (and of younger people with sufficient knowledge and understanding) to make their own decisions about accepting or not accepting medical interventions, even against medical advice. In my experience, critics of autonomy tend to be at least somewhat religious (the religious attitude studies cited above bear that out) and though not necessarily as doctrinaire as those who think rational suicide is a sin, the concept still disturbs them at some fundamental level. They also tend to argue that current British (or English) law and the Swiss Option are a satisfactory compromise because the law acts as a deterrent and the Director of Public Prosecutions can be relied on to be merciful.

The other slippery slope is the one onto which, it is alleged, large numbers of people with physical and mental disabilities, who have never expressed any desire for deliverance from their conditions, will be encouraged to enter by family members, stigma and social pressure, or by the State that spends so much money on their care and is always looking for economies. In this scenario, the disabled will not so much walk or crawl reluctantly onto the slope but will be pushed onto it willy-nilly in their wheelchairs, reaching out in vain for ethical and legal handholds as they accelerate down towards the final precipice. This scenario is invoked by both religious critics and non-religious ones like the right-of-centre, atheist, gay, libertarian journalist Douglas Murray – a man I greatly admire for his brave defence of our hard-won freedom to criticize all religions, including Islam. For Murray, the 'slippery slope' is evidently a daily concern.[134] "I think continually about this" he writes. "Perhaps this will become the dominant vision of life in Britain…. But I cannot wish for it. There's the slippery slope, the uncertain old who may feel pressured, the pathetic cases of depressed teenagers choosing death, and the shift in meaning

---

[134] https://www.spectator.co.uk/2015/08/the-atheist-case-against-assisted
-dying/

it brings to life as well as death." Despite his atheism, Murray seems to feel that life must have some sort of cosmic purpose and meaning beyond our relationships with our fellow-humans – living, dead or yet to be born.[135] As he notes, most religions do offer such cosmic purposes but I suspect that many or even most of his fellow-unbelievers sympathise with the view of the philosopher Sir Isaiah Berlin that "As for the meaning of life, I do not believe that it has any: I do not at all ask what it is, for I suspect it has none, and this is a source of great comfort to me — we make of it what we can, and that is all there is about it."[136] However, Murray also worries about the slow but steady increase in Dutch and Belgian deaths by voluntary euthanasia (our opponents often leave out that crucial adjective) and their equivalents in states where deliverance is legal. I will deal with that objection first.

One explanation for the increase is surely the same one that accounts for the gradual – even hesitant – adoption of many other new ideas, technologies and freedoms: including, I suppose, the relatively recent freedom to come out as a gay journalist without any serious legal or professional consequences. Take cremation, for a particularly relevant example. Although it was customary in many Eastern cultures, it was illegal in Britain (give or take the odd heretic) until late in the 19th century. As with voluntary euthanasia in the 1930s, a small group of the Great and Good in Victorian Britain (which, like the founders of the Voluntary Euthanasia Society, also included a royal surgeon) formed a society in 1874 to promote cremation but it was not until 1902 that it was legalized in the face of much opposition, later than in Italy and France but before Portugal in 1920 and well

---

[135] Murray D. The strange death of Europe: immigration, identity and Islam. London, Bloomsbury 2018, 266 and *passim.*

[136] Cited in Cartwright J. new.spectator.co.uk/2015/10/fear-loneliness-and–nostalgia-a-return-to-johannesburg/

before Greece in 2016. In 1905, over 99% of British families buried their dead. By 1960, that had fallen to 40% and it is now around 30%. Some religions – including Orthodox Judaism and Islam – still prohibit it. In Greece, the Orthodox church tried to block its recent legalisation and apparently threatens to excommunicate those who would ignore its pronouncements. Today, there may even be a financial incentive to cremate rather than bury but though cremation aroused very high emotions a century ago, few people now seem to worry about it and those with strong feelings are entirely free to choose burial.[137]

For those who are concerned about safeguards against abuse – which includes everyone I know in the debate – another relevant analogy is the way in which motor cars were hesitantly allowed onto British roads. As every schoolchild knows, they were at first limited to 4 mph and had to be preceded by a man carrying a red flag. That may have been a sensible precaution, especially on country roads where horse-drawn wagons moved slowly and cantering or galloping horses gave plenty of audible warning but the precaution was quickly relaxed. Soon, anyone could get a driving licence without even a test (my mother, an anxious and over-cautious driver, was theoretically free to drive heavy lorries) but in the 1930s, driving tests were introduced. In other words, checks and balances were adjusted as experience of the new – and dangerous – technology increased, for in 1930, there were over 7000 deaths on British roads. By 1950, with many more cars, that dropped to 5000 and despite an eight-fold increase in car ownership since then, a combination of drink-driving laws and better cars, roads and trauma care has taken the figure to well below 2000 for the last several years. The same gradual process can be seen with everything from unregulated

---

[137] As – for entirely non–religious reasons – I would. Cremation seems such a waste of gas and I like the idea of being usefully reincarnated as a tree following a woodland burial.

activities such as foreign travel, extreme sports and sales of avocado and garlic to heavily regulated ones like voting rights, contraception and the right of heretics to become Members of Parliament. (Catholics in 1829, Jews in 1858, atheists in 1888.) It happens regularly when things that were previously unthinkable or unsayable – or just not on most people's radar – become matters of public debate.

Is it surprising if more and more patients suffering from unpleasant and intractable or terminal conditions, in jurisdictions from the Netherlands to Oregon and Australia, have taken advantage of the freedom the law allows them to choose the time and manner of their deaths in the way that many doctors are able to do? There are obvious advantages to be had from dying peacefully, predictably and in the company of loved ones - perhaps to the sound of one's favourite music after a last taste of one's favourite food and wine.[138] And without anxiety about frightening terminal symptoms such as fighting for breath and palpitations; without being confused, hallucinating and barely conscious for several days because of high doses of morphine and sedatives; or of diminishing the dignity of the final farewell and the carefully chosen last words by an all-too-noticeable attack of vomiting or faecal incontinence. Those who, for whatever reasons, prefer the natural, drawn-out but often unpredictable version are free to choose it. Palliative care and hospices exist in part to cater for their tastes. Not everyone wants a planned and medicalised death and far more people evidently prefer not to think too

---

[138] My copy of Dr W. Munk's 'Euthanasia: or, Medical Treatment in Aid of an Easy Death' (London. Longmans, Green. 1887) has a whole chapter about choosing the right wine for the dying. He recommends Tokay as "often more acceptable than any other wine...It is best given with cream". The book is actually about terminal care and does not encourage the accelerating of death, though Munk recognises that such practices are "very prevalent in France and Germany and...not unknown in this country".

much – or at all – about death but the rise in popularity of medicalised death is no more surprising than the growing popularity of cremation, or of major medical involvement at the other end of life, as discussed in Chapter 15.

Murray also compares the increase in deliverance in countries that allow it to the increase in abortion that followed its decriminalization in Britain in 1968. It is true that within a few years, more women were having abortions that some people who were not opposed to reform had expected and some of those people think the number should be reduced. For others, abortion remains the equivalent of murder and therefore all abortions are not merely wrong but irredeemably wicked as well. There are two responses to the comparison with abortion. The first regards it as one of the rights of women that have been recently acquired (historically speaking) after aeons of male dominance. *Machismo* was a necessary and universal survival trait in competing tribal societies but it is less universally important for our survival now and less appropriate for a more peaceful and gender-equal society. Most anti-abortionists were the spiritual heirs of the people who had opposed contraception with equal fervour a generation or two earlier. Some were the same people. Some supposedly beneficial social changes – 'progressive' or not – have disadvantages as well as benefits. The abortion laws have been blamed for the failure of European societies to breed at replacement levels, but falling pregnancy rates are a feature of all societies that enable women to obtain education, employment, contraception and a measure of freedom from the control of their husbands (and clerics). The legalisation of abortion is just one factor and a fairly small one.

The second is to note the embarrassed silence of anti-abortionists when one points out a major paradox of protests and political opposition that stem from a belief that abortion is wicked, that it should be reduced (or become once more illegal, as it still is in much of South America) and that human life begins at fertilization when the unique genetic combination that will produce a new and unique human being takes place. The following paragraph or two may seem a little tangential but bear with me, because abortion is also very relevant to the arguments of one of the most emotive and visible opposition groups – the disability lobby – which I will discuss shortly. To be morally consistent, anti-abortionists should really be complaining and demonstrating not outside abortion clinics but outside family planning clinics that recommend and insert – as nearly all do – various kinds of Intrauterine Contraceptive Device (the IUD or 'coil'). It has been beyond doubt since the early 1980s that although IUDs can prevent pregnancy by preventing fertilization, an important additional mechanism is that they also destroy tiny embryos *after* fertilization and also wipe them off the wall of the uterus if they get as far as implantation.[139] In other words, they are abortifacients. If British abortion figures applied to the whole 500 million-plus population of the EU, there would be about 2 million abortions annually. If the 150 million women throughout the world who have IUDs have just one early IUD-induced abortion annually – which is almost certainly an underestimate – their 150 million-plus abortions completely dwarf that figure.

If one abortion is bad, then 150 million must surely be not only 150 million times worse but also 75 times worse than 2 million, yet anti abortionists – including successive Popes – rarely mention the paradox. The reason is that they know that hardly anyone cares about the moral status of something that is barely visible to the naked eye but they cannot admit that without admitting that in practice, *they* don't seem to care much about it either; and that therefore

---

[139] Brewer C. The mortal coil. BMJ 2012; 345 doi: http://dx.doi.org/10.1136/bmj.e7551

'murdering a potential Beethoven' doesn't matter provided it's only a little one. Once they concede that early abortion isn't something that arouses their anger much, or at all, the argument changes from whether abortion is right or wrong to the stage at which it starts to become an ethical concern. That, in turn, becomes an argument about pain, awareness, neurodevelopment, memory, and even aesthetics but since nobody remembers the unpleasant business of being squeezed through the birth canal or – if a Jewish or Muslim male – of being circumcised without anaesthesia a few days after birth, the 'argument from pain' (dramatized in the 1970s by anti-abortionists in a film called 'The Silent Scream') falls very flat.[140]

This brings me to the first of Douglas Murray's concerns – the people 'who may feel pressured' by the mere existence of legalized deliverance, among whom, he implies, are the disabled as well as those who are merely old. You may still feel that the abortion arguments are tangential to the debate about deliverance but though it is not often mentioned by them, abortion is also particularly relevant to that section of the disability lobby which campaigns very visibly and loudly against deliverance. It is composed mainly of people with severe and often congenital physical disabilities and some (but by no means all) of their non-disabled advocates. It is the principal owner and promoter of the argument that if deliverance is legalized, disabled people will be put under strong pressure to agree to die, though I do not think they have ever produced a single example of the medically-assisted death of a conscious, adult patient arising from such pressure. There

---

[140] Though not quite as flat as the book 'Babies for Burning', which absurdly claimed that the fat from aborted foetuses was being systematically used for making soap – a claim exploded by the Sunday Times. The human foetus has hardly any fat until the last few weeks of pregnancy and most abortions are done between 8 and 12 weeks when the foetus may be no more than 2cm in length.

are people with severe disabilities among the active members of right-to-die societies, who demand that they should not be denied the choices that are open to the 'abled'. A very small number of relatively young severely disabled British residents have indeed chosen the Swiss option. Others have chosen self-deliverance and sometimes succeeded, including a young paraplegic who died inside his specially-adapted house after deliberately setting fire to it, other methods having failed. It is possible that a modest increase in cases of deliverance may occur but, as Ian Brassington pointed out in his criticism of Yuill, a belief by individuals or society that it is a good thing not to suffer from multiple sclerosis or quadriplegia is entirely compatible with providing good and constantly improving care to people with disabilities and to encourage them to integrate with the abled majority where possible and vice versa. (Similarly, one can question the large-scale immigration of people with very different cultures and customs, as Murray does, while insisting that those who have arrived must be treated well and helped and encouraged to integrate with the host community.)

Yet a far bigger theoretical threat to the peace of mind and self-esteem of the disabled is one that they seem to have dealt with easily and with very little public debate. It is one thing to argue that disabled people have rights to good treatment or social service provision, easy access to public spaces and to be protected against discrimination. Who would disagree with that? It is quite another thing to suggest – as some disability activists sometimes appear to do – that no mother or father should try to avoid having a disabled child, and that profoundly and congenitally deaf children or children with Down syndrome or severe spina bifida, for example, should be just as desirable, in prospect, as children without these conditions. There are arguments – mainly religious – against both pre-natal testing and abortion but they do not deter the large majority of prospective parents in all countries where testing is available. Even in countries with laws that permit abortion only for very restricted reasons, the prospect of giving birth to a seriously disabled child is usually one of those reasons. As I discuss in more detail in Chapter 15, developments in antenatal and pre-implantation diagnosis have almost abolished the birth of children with some major types of disability that were once common, notably in Iceland. If that kind of discrimination against the disabled has upset the disability lobby, they have kept rather quiet about it. There is some debate, but not much and no campaigning that remotely matches their other concerns. One Icelandic geneticist was quoted as saying: "I don't think there's anything wrong with aspiring to have healthy children, but how far we should go in seeking those goals is a fairly complicated decision". For most mothers and families, it is evidently not very complicated in practice.

One other slippery slope – allowing people not only to choose deliverance in early dementia before they lose Capacity but also to request and receive it at some stage after they have lost it – will be discussed in Chapter 14. As we have seen, something like it already exists – sometimes voluntary but mostly involuntary – in a legal twilight zone but many people seem reluctant to discuss the implications of what happens in that zone every day and night in Britain and everywhere else with health services. By mentioning the topic at all, my aim is no more than to start and encourage a conversation about a very difficult problem. However, even moderate familiarity with treating, nursing or just caring for people with dementia makes it difficult to argue that the severely demented never experience severe suffering. Furthermore, when people as diverse as Quebec nurses and caregivers and Conservative journalists like Matthew Parris think the problem is worth researching and writing about, I don't feel I need to apologise for doing the same. Nevertheless, the overwhelming priority in

Britain is for laws that will make it unnecessary for any patient or family member to say to a doctor – as many do and many more think – 'you wouldn't allow a dog to suffer like this'. My basic argument for focusing on dementia in the wider debate about deliverance is that the concept of suffering needs to include the existential and anticipatory kinds to which dogs – perhaps happily for them – are, as far as we know, immune. I shall be very pleased but still slightly surprised if even limited British deliverance legislation reaches the statute book in my expected lifetime. If at some stage that law is passed and later expanded, we know that electorates can change their minds, though so far, no electorate has repealed such laws[141] and Dutch doctors are still the world's most trusted and highly regarded ("Out of all the countries we found surveys for, it was Dutch patients who found it hardest to fault their doctors, especially GPs".[142]) It also appears that a large majority of the Dutch electorate both strongly support the existing law and practice and are willing to accept some cautious expansion that extends the concept of autonomy to the treatment of dead personalities, just as cremation extended it to the treatment of dead bodies. There is, of course, one more slippery slope but it is slippery with faeces, urine and – not infrequently – pus from bedsores that in very thin and frail old people can sometimes eat through as far as the underlying bone. For many people with early dementia contemplating their future, these are important additional reasons for not wanting to risk getting onto the slope that most concerns them.

A final point. There are many laws and regulations aimed at minimizing the risk of a wide range of harms to citizens

---

[141] The reversal of the first legislation that permitted MAiD – in Australia's Northern Territory in 1996 – was overturned on a technicality by the Federal Parliament, not by the NT's voters or legislators.

[142] Kmietovicz Z. R.E.S.P.E.C.T.—why doctors are still getting enough of it. BMJ 2002 v.324 (7328); 2002. Jan 5 PMC1121933

at all stages of life. We rightly expect those laws to reduce the risks that are inherent in most human activities but few people expect them to reduce the risks to absolute zero. If that were the case, nobody would be allowed to take a train or a plane, since fatal accidents still happen occasionally even in the most technologically advanced countries. Still less would anybody be allowed to drive a car. Despite rigorous checks – which are a routine professional reflex as well as an implicit legal requirement – surgeons still occasionally operate on the wrong limb or organ, or leave swabs or instruments inside the patient and even after perfectly performed surgery, people occasionally die unexpectedly but we do not therefore outlaw surgery. Similar disasters occur when patients receive the wrong medicines or the wrong doses, or die from rare side-effects. The laws and regulations aimed at safeguarding the process of deliverance do not need to be better than their equivalents for other irreversible interventions. However, unlike decisions about high-risk surgical and pharmacological treatments, which often need to be made quickly, planning by patients for situations that might lead them to request deliverance often begins – and should begin – well before any signs of disease appear. As with all regulations, there is a balance to be struck between protecting patients (and professionals) against mistakes, misunderstandings or malice and making the procedures so burdensome and protracted that patients cannot access deliverance at all or have to experience significant periods of severe suffering before obtaining it. There is remarkably little evidence that laws allowing patients to choose medical aid in dying are abused.

10

Leave it to Palliative Care
and Hospices?

This is a short chapter, because palliative and hospice care really have very little to offer patients with moderate or severe dementia. It would have been even shorter but for one very curious fact. Namely, that although there are British palliative care physicians who support deliverance, I was unable, while writing the book, to find a single one at consultant level who was willing to give me a supportive statement on – or even off – the record, and I thought it necessary to add a short section about this truly remarkable silence.

In part, the shortness reflects the plentiful evidence that palliative care professionals themselves are confused about their role in dementia. Even in Norway, a very civilized and extremely prosperous country with exemplary health and social services, a study tellingly titled "A painful experience of limited understanding: healthcare professionals' experiences with palliative care of people with severe dementia in Norwegian nursing homes" found that experienced staff faced distressing challenges "related to 'reading' the patients' suffering, coming up short despite occasional success, handing the patients over to strangers, and disagreeing on the patients' best interests… Occasionally, they succeeded and were able to calm the patients, but they often [failed with] pain relief and coping with behavioural symptoms, such as aggression and rejection of care".[143] Wanting to collaborate with patients' families to "ensure the best possible palliative care", they often encountered "difficult situations when they disagreed with the family on the patients' best interests".

The mission statement of Palliative Care is generally something like: 'helping people to live until they die'. Since 'living' means different things to different people, this means, according to the International Association for Hospice and Palliative care, that staff need, at some point, to have discussions with patients along the following lines:

"Introduce the discussion (e.g. We need to talk about your current problems and our goals for your care).

Find out what they understand (e.g. 'Tell me in your own words what you understand about your illness at the moment. Don't worry if you cannot remember medical terms.').

Find out what they expect (e.g. 'Tell me what you see happening with this illness in the future....Tell me what things are important for you, perhaps things you've not mentioned before...Tell me what you don't like about what we've done or said – we won't be upset or angry, I promise you.')".[144]

Such enquiries are obviously appropriate and desirable for patients, even of limited years or intelligence, who can recall past events and anticipate future ones but they are unhelpful when both memory and anticipation no longer exist and even a very simple conversation may be impossible. In cases of

---

[143] Midtbust MH, Alnes RE, Gjengedal E, Lykkeslet E. A painful experience of limited understanding: healthcare professionals' experiences with palliative care of people with severe dementia in Norwegian nursing homes. BMC Palliat Care. 2018 Feb 13;17(1):25. doi: 10.1186/s12904–018–0282–8.

[144] https://hospicecare.com/what–we–do/publications/getting–started/6–principles–of–palliative–care/

terminal cancer, for example, when patients are too confused to answer questions, they may have indicated their preferences before becoming confused and what the family wants will often be what the patient wanted but this is evidently not always the case with dementia. When doctors from Holland visited the prestigious St Christopher's Hospice in London and interviewed staff members, they identified "five themes.. home/homelike, community, consideration of others, link with outside world, and privacy".[145] Again, fine for patients with reasonably full awareness, even if they are not 'terminal' but of what interest are these concerns to a bed-bound patient with advanced dementia who does not interact with other patients, often seems frightened of the nurses and does not recognize close family members? In advanced dementia, one can't talk about using the dying period to restore or repair relationships, find unexpected pleasures, deal with spiritual concerns, do bucket lists or try to hang on for the birth of a grandchild. No wonder the Norwegian palliative care staff found the experience 'painful'.

In any case, patients with advanced dementia "often fail to receive palliative care" and although "[b]arriers to the delivery of palliative care for people with dementia have been studied for more than a decade, yet at present, there is a lack of consensus in practice".[146] Note that all these references are to recent studies. They are not about practices and attitudes that are no longer relevant to modern palliative care. Many patients with dementia are old enough to have acquired other degenerative diseases as well and as we have seen, pain on movement and even at rest

---

[145] West E, Onwuteaka–Philipsen , Philipsen H2, Higginson IJ, Pasman HRW. "Keep All Thee 'Til the End": Reclaiming the Lifeworld for Patients in the Hospice Setting. Omega (Westport). 2017 Jan 1:30222817697040. doi: 10.1177/0030222817697040.

[146] Erel M, Marcus EL, Dekeyser–Ganz F. Barriers to palliative care for advanced dementia: a scoping review. Ann Palliat Med. 2017 Oct;6(4):365–379. doi: 10.21037/apm.2017.06.13.

is both common and often inadequately treated. It should not specifically need a palliative care team to persuade the staff of nursing homes to take pain more seriously and to teach them how best to maximise the desirable effects of opiates, for example, while minimising their undesirable ones such as constipation, thus reducing the need for procedures like the manual evacuation of faeces that are greatly disliked by both patients and doctors.

The only mention of palliative care in the Key Findings summary of the 2016 report of Alzheimer's Disease International refers to the "significant gaps in research into…the cost-effectiveness of…advanced care planning and palliative care approaches".[147] An earlier paragraph urges that "healthcare should be continuous, holistic and person-centred, treating the whole person according to [patients'] values and preferences". We know that for many patients, the 'values and preferences' expressed when they were still able to make decisions about their future management mean the rejection of all efforts to prolong their lives and the hope that they will die as soon as possible. We also know that where dementia is concerned, most palliative care teams cannot deliver on that because they are constitutionally, philosophically and often doctrinally opposed to that particular type of person-centredness.

Let us return now to the deafening silence of palliative care consultants who may support some sort of Medical Assistance in Dying but are clearly too frightened to say so publicly. In 2012, Dr. Sam Ahmedzai, who was, at that time, the Professor of Palliative Care at Sheffield University, wrote a short opinion piece for the British Medical Journal, describing his "journey from anti- to pro-assisted dying".[148] His views evidently changed

---

[147] https://www.alz.co.uk/research/worldalzheimerreport2016sheet.pdf [accessed 28 Feb 2018]

[148] Ahmedzai S. My journey from anti- to pro-assisted dying BMJ 2012; 9 July 2012 345:e4592

following visits to Oregon and the Netherlands, where he saw good palliative care coexisting fairly amicably with deliverance. "It is patronizing" he wrote "to say that a few people should suffer unbearable distress and indignity because palliative care preaches that it values all lives – regardless of how meaningless they have become to their owners", adding: "it is hypocritical to deny competent patients who are acknowledged to be dying the right to die in the manner of their choosing".

The following year, at the AGM of Healthcare Professionals for Assisted Dying (a group that supports the aims of Dignity in Dying) Professor Ahmedzai repeated these views. He emphasised the need to continue clinical innovation but seemed to be advocating philosophical and ethical innovation as well, in order to provide a more patient-focused approach at the end-of-life, including the option of deliverance. I met him for the first time at a meeting around 2016 and we had a friendly discussion. When I asked him why he had not even replied to my request for a short contribution to the 2015 collection of essays – *I'll See Myself Out, Thank You* – that I co-edited, he explained that his membership of a NHS 'best practice' guidelines committee restricted his freedom.

Recently, I was told by one of my senior contacts in palliative care (who I won't embarrass by identifying) that Professor Ahmedzai had now retired and would surely be willing to talk. I immediately emailed him but once again got no reply. Not surprisingly, I interpreted this as the result of pressure on him not to rock the palliative boat. Apart from the inappropriateness and limitations of palliative and hospice care for advanced dementia, the well-documented over-representation of religious doctors in British palliative care[149] means that many of them

---

[149] Seale C. The role of doctors' religious faith and ethnicity in taking ethically controversial decisions during end-of-life care. J Med Ethics 2010 Nov;36(11):677–82

must find it very difficult or even impossible to accept patient autonomy in this most crucial and fundamental area. I thought that the palliative care establishment had been twisting Professor Ahmedzai's arm to keep quiet, because I knew they were doing that to other would-be dissenters. It is statistically unlikely that every single UK palliative care consultant holds views about deliverance that are at variance with the views of some 90% of the British public. I thought it equally unlikely that Professor Ahmedzai is the only palliative care consultant who agrees with the significant percentage of British doctors in all other specialties who do support deliverance of some kind. If there really are no dissident voices in palliative care, that would be very worrying indeed, for it would suggest that they are very unlike their colleagues in jurisdictions such as Oregon, the Netherlands, Canada and Colombia. And even more unlike their Belgian palliative care colleagues, who were the main drivers of deliverance legislation. These apparently doctrinaire and monolithic views therefore make many British palliative care physicians, in *some* very important respects, unfit – or at any rate, much less than ideal – for a medical specialty that deals every day with human beings holding diverse views on one of the most important stages of life. However, at the last possible moment to include it in the book, I had another conversation with Professor Ahmedzai that clarified his position. He contacted me because of my published responses to an article in the BMJ in which I had mentioned his name and my suspicions about arm-twisting.

The article was a Canadian version of Professor Ahmedzai's 2012 story in the British Medical Journal about how the author had changed his mind about MAID.[150] Like Professor Ahmedzai, Dr Sandy Buchman is a palliative care specialist but he is also

---

[150] Buchman S. Why I decided to provide assisted dying: it is truly patient centred care. BMJ 2019;364:l412

the president-elect of the Canadian Medical Association – the Canadian equivalent of the BMA. Interestingly, his first voluntary euthanasia patient was another physician: "Gordon Froggatt was a 79 year old professor emeritus of medicine and a cardiologist. He gave me written permission to share his story because he believed in the option of medical assistance in dying and wanted the profession and the public to learn from his experience." Even more interesting and relevant to this book was the diagnosis. "He had advanced Parkinson's disease and very early Lewy body dementia. He understood his fate all too well. He had become unable to feed and toilet himself or even to roll over on his own in bed. He had profound uncontrollable torso and head shaking. As a proud family man and respected member of the medical community, he found the loss of independence and inability to care for himself unacceptable. He had sunk into a deep depression. He received compassionate care and treatment from his geriatric psychiatrist, his devoted neurologist, and his family physician. Finally, I provided his palliative care. He knew MAID had just become legal in Canada, and he asked me if we could talk about it. When I agreed, it was as though a huge burden was lifted from his shoulders."

Canada's MAID laws do not put a 6-month or 12-month time-limit on what constitutes 'terminal' illness and the course of Parkinsonism, even when advanced, is not easy to predict with confidence but his death was judged to be "reasonably foreseeable" by his neurologist, meaning that "his medical conditions ultimately will end in death, without specifying an exact life expectancy or prognosis but implying that he was terminally ill". His psychiatrist reviewed him and confirmed that he had Mental Capacity. He also found that he was "no longer…depressed", though I think that 'understandable misery' would probably have been a more accurate diagnosis and a better description of his earlier state and that it understandably disappeared, along with the "huge burden", when Dr Buchman agreed to put an end to his misery. No antidepressant works as instantaneously as that.

Because of the severe shaking affecting his head and hands (presumably the reason he could not feed himself) Dr Froggatt exercised the choice of 99.9% of Canadian MAID recipients to have their lethal medication administered intravenously by a doctor, rather than drinking it. Midazolam (a Valium-type drug widely used for endoscopic procedures) was injected to produce unconsciousness. Then the anaesthetic drug Propofol (which unintentionally caused the death of Michael Jackson when given without proper anaesthetic supervision) was injected at a dose that would eventually stop his breathing. To make absolutely sure and to minimise the interval between the first injection and death, which was "a few minutes", a curare-type drug was then injected that quickly paralysed the respiratory muscles. "He died the most peaceful death I had ever witnessed, in the arms of his daughter, in his own home, surrounded by people who loved him. I realised, then, that this procedure was the most patient-centred service I could offer. I alleviated his suffering in a way that wasn't possible through any other means. This experience exemplified for me the reason I went into medicine: to alleviate suffering. I know that's what I did for Gordon."

At our meeting, Professor Ahmedzai explained that he was still constrained by membership of the committee but confirmed that he has not changed his views and will resume his important part in the debate when he is free to do so. He also confirmed both my assumption that he is not the only senior British palliative care physician to be in favour of MAID and my strong suspicion that such dissidents have been too 'intimidated' (his choice of word) by the palliative care establishment to join him on his journey out of the palliative closet — a suspicion that had been angrily denounced by several members of that establishment in published responses to Dr Buchman. Perhaps he knew even more than he told me because on March 21st, the BMJ published an article by five *anonymous* senior palliative care physicians[151] titled 'We risk our careers if we discuss assisted dying, say UK palliative care consultants'.

"All of us", they wrote, "have been rebutted or stifled from airing this topic. We believe that there may be many more colleagues – especially trainees and early career consultants – who do not share the views of the officers of the APM [Association of Palliative Medicine] but we suspect they are intimidated and inhibited from openly sharing the views that we have put forward here... There is no concession to the possibility that other doctors practising high quality and ethical specialist palliative medicine may hold an alternative opinion or just want to hear about different options." As they say in courtroom dramas, 'I rest my case'.

---

[151] https://blogs.bmj.com/bmj/2019/03/21/we-risk-our-careers-if-we-discuss-assisted-dying-say-uk-palliative-care-consultants/

11

Families in Conflict

One day, I was travelling to my primary school on the usual bus, which also passed a local cemetery. The woman in the next seat was joined by a man who had just got on at the cemetery stop. They knew each other and the man explained that he had been visiting the cemetery to put some flowers on his wife's grave. "I don't know why I do it", he said. "We were always arguing. I never bought flowers for her when she was alive". I thus learned early in life that death and grief are not simple and straightforward matters. This kind of ambivalent, contradictory, confused and possibly guilt-laden thought and behaviour is also very common among family members faced with decisions about end-of-life (EOL) care in advanced dementia, especially when resuscitation is the issue. Even when families are reasonably harmonious, a review of this problem found that "denial, stigma, and conflicting family perceptions of what constitutes quality of life and a 'good death' are barriers to engaging in EOL discussions".[152] The authors

---

[152] Carlozzi NE, Downing NR, McCormack MK, et al. New measures to capture end of life concerns in Huntington disease: Meaning and Purpose and Concern with Death and Dying from HDQLIFE (a patient reported outcomes measurement system). *Quality of life research : an international journal of quality of life aspects of treatment, care and rehabilitation.* 2016;25(10):2403–2415. doi:10.1007/s11136–016–1354–y.

also noted:"..that talking about these issues can be uncomfortable for both the patient and the provider, that [patients]...often do not discuss these concerns with physicians, that physicians often neglect to initiate discussions about EOL options with patients, and that this has been recognized as a priority area for...clinical care". The dementia, in this case, was due to Huntington's rather than Alzheimer's Disease but in both conditions, the end-states and the EOL concerns are identical.

The marked ambivalence of medical and nursing staff about resuscitation and active treatment that was summarised in Chapters 6 and 7 is just as evident among family members and an equally wide range of views exists. For example, a recent study that asked family members who had experience of a death from advanced dementia about the "acceptability of an advance directive that limits food and liquids" in that situation – in other words, about facilitating death from dehydration – found that "all participants in our focus group stated that an advance directive that would include withdrawal of food and liquids would not conflict with their religious beliefs". However, when asked how they would respond if a patient with such an advance directive then verbally or nonverbally expressed a desire for food or drink, "everybody indicated that such a person should receive help with eating or drinking...although it is against the wishes he expressed in his advance directive". Unless generous sedation is given when food and fluids are withdrawn, it is not difficult to see why both family members and health professionals may find it hard to accept such directives. In some cases, the directive was evidently honoured but one family member stated: "The last three days were the worst for me, watching her starve to death. It happened two years ago and I am just getting the image out of my head".

It is doubtful that three days of peaceful drug-induced sleep would have been anywhere near as traumatic for the family. That view is reinforced by one of the very few studies that examined levels of apparent distress in patients with advanced dementia when artificial nutrition was either not started or was withdrawn.[153] The qualifier 'apparent' is needed because by this stage, the patients were unable to communicate their feelings (or, it would seem, anything coherent at all) and adequate nutrition and hydration could not be maintained because "the patients scarcely or no longer ate or drank". Conclusions had to be drawn from observable behaviour such as restlessness, facial expressions, breathing difficulties and "negative vocalisation". Unsurprisingly, sleeping patients seemed to be much less distressed than those who remained awake but despite apparently generous levels of analgesic and sedative medication, the majority appeared to have little sleep until near the end. Nevertheless, for most patients, levels of distress gradually diminished once nutritional assistance was withdrawn but even though that withdrawal was clearly intended to avoid prolongation of the terminal phase or even to accelerate it, some patients continued to receive fluids and the more fluid they received, the longer they lived. Over half died during the first five days but 24 of the 174 were still alive six weeks later. As well as severe dementia (Alzheimer-type in 43%; average age 85) about half the patients had developed an acute illness such as pneumonia or urinary infection. Consistent with the decision to withdraw or withhold artificial nutrition, antibiotics and most other active treatments were either not started or discontinued. Patients received standard oral hygiene and treatment to avoid or control bedsores but the fact that some received significant and life-prolonging quantities of fluid by mouth seems to indicate significant levels of ambivalence in the medical and nursing staff.

---

[153] Pasman HR, Onwuteaka–Philipsen BD, Kriegsman DM, et al Discomfort in nursing home patients with severe dementia in whom artificial nutrition and hydration is forgone. Arch Intern Med. 2005 Aug 8–22;165(15):1729–35.

Another motivation for actively treating and resuscitating patients who might not have wanted such attention was mentioned by one member of a focus group. "Keeping people alive is not because it is best for them but because it is best for us. My husband at his end, for months, I could still touch him, I could put my arm around him, I could get in the bed with him. And I told a nurse, it means a lot to me. I do not know if it means anything for him. 'And it means a lot for him too', she said. We cannot let go.'"

I find it difficult to decide my own response to her statement. One can understand the desire of a spouse or partner to retain the possibility of physical contact even when a two-way conversation becomes impossible. On the other hand, I am not sure that I would want to stay alive and use up valuable health resources for encounters not far removed from going to bed with someone while very drunk (or after swallowing a drink spiked with a date-rape drug) and waking up without any recollection of the night's activities, however pleasant and memorable they may have been for the other party.

Even when patients have made it clear that they would prefer not to be treated, the pressure from some family members to 'do something' can be hard to resist. Sometimes, a single dissenting (and often unrealistic) family member can play on the guilt and uncertainty of other members when a DNR decision is in the balance. In one case known to me, the dissenting member eventually changed her mind but by that time, inappropriate resuscitation had ensured that her mother spent many more months in a care home with extremely poor quality of life before she died from another acute illness. Many living wills nominate a proxy – usually a spouse or other close family member – to make treatment decisions when the patient can no longer do so. Registering a Health Care Power of Attorney strengthens that arrangement but a recent controlled study from Quebec found that even when elderly but reasonably healthy citizens were encouraged and assisted to document their preferences for treatment or non-treatment and to communicate those preferences to their chosen proxy, "the intervention... had little effect on proxies' ability to predict them".[154] In the event of severe dementia, about 90% of the 265 mainly Catholic subjects would refuse intravenous antibiotics for any condition, or surgery for an acutely inflamed gall–bladder (a notoriously painful emergency) yet the proxies would have chosen these interventions twice as often, as they would have done for tube-feeding.

Opponents of MAID frequently claim that dementia patients could be coerced into requesting deliverance, or be deprived of resuscitation, by pressure from family members worried that their potential inheritance is being steadily reduced by nursing home fees. Living wills and advance decisions to refuse treatment made well in advance of dementia, and the use of Health Care Powers of Attorney (discussed later) are two obvious ways of minimising that risk, which in any case only arises in countries that do not provide free nursing home care, or demand only a proportion of the patient's pension or sickness benefits. In reality, dementia patients currently experience a great deal of coercion and pressure to remain alive when they would either definitely or probably prefer to be dead. Apart from the various doctors' dilemmas previously discussed and the financial incentives in fee-per-item health services to resuscitate patients and to keep beds filled, patients can be subjected by family members to financial pressures to remain alive that are just as objectionable as pressures to shorten their lives would be. Here is an example reported to me by someone who is close to the family involved. A few unimportant details have been

---

[154] Bravo G, Trottier L, Arcand M, et al. Promoting advance care planning among community–based older adults: A randomized controlled trial. Patient Educ Couns 2016: 99, 1785–95

changed to preserve anonymity but I suspect that the story is not an uncommon one.

Victor is now in his 40s and has never been in a long-term relationship. He did not complete his university degree and subsequently drifted from one relatively low-paid job to another. He has often received social security benefits and spends a lot of time in front of his computer screen. An only child, he did not have a good relationship with either of his parents and they divorced when he was 16. For about 15 years after Victor left home to go to university, his mother saw him only infrequently but when she developed Alzheimer's, Victor saw an opportunity. Once his mother could no longer live safely on her own, he moved back to the family home as the primary carer. Five years into her dementia, his mother sits in a chair for most of the day, is occasionally incontinent but is apathetic rather than agitated. Nevertheless, neighbours often hear Victor shouting at her. She never made a living will and her views on remaining alive in a state of dementia are not known but she would be unusual if she wanted to be kept alive at all costs. Helpers from the social services visit regularly to share the tasks of care. Victor has control of his mother's finances, which include a reasonable pension and various sickness benefits. He spends most of the day glued to his computer. When his mother dies, he will inherit the house but will lose his mother's income. On several occasions, his mother has been admitted to hospital with life-threatening conditions. The physicians question the benefits and appropriateness of resuscitation and intensive care but every time, Victor insists that 'everything must be done' and the physicians have so far found it easier to agree than to refuse.

I end this chapter with a short account of how family conflicts played out in a rather public way in the case of the writer Katherine Whitehorn when her friend and fellow-journalist Polly Toynbee wrote about Katherine's dementia in the Guardian ('Katharine Whitehorn would rather die than live like this').[155]

"Katharine is now 90, living in a care home, suffering from Alzheimer's, with little understanding left, no knowledge of where she is or why. She often doesn't recognise people, can no longer read and curiously sometimes talks in French, not a language she knew particularly well: she will never read or understand this article. In other words, she is not herself. Her old self would not recognise herself in this other being who sits in the care home dayroom. What or who she has become is a difficult philosophical question, but she is no longer Katharine Whitehorn as was."

Polly noted Katherine's views on one of the basic causes of the problem. "Oregon at least shows the way forward for dealing with a problem that is not brought about by too little health care, but almost by too much – by our ability to keep people alive long after they would once have served their term." On the basic philosophical problem, she wrote "Surely the real Katharine Whitehorn, the one in her right mind, is custodian of herself, arbiter of what or who is her real self and when to discard an empty husk? (And no, this personal custodianship has no bearing on the rights of disabled people.)"

Katherine's son Bernard Lyall responded in a piece titled 'My mother favours assisted dying. Now she has dementia I'm not sure I agree'.[156] "Kath had argued for the right to die, has a living will, and would have been horrified to see herself like this." he wrote. "Three years ago, gripped by pneumonia, she thought she was dying, and was quite relaxed, and touchingly grateful for all that life had brought her. But now the power to let her

---

[155] https://www.theguardian.com/commentisfree/2018/may/29/assisted–dying-katharine-whitehorn-alzheimers

[156] https://www.theguardian.com/commentisfree/2018/jul/01/katharine-whitehorn-dementia-alzheimers

go has fallen to me, it's not so simple."Things weren't made any easier by Katherine's reluctance in the early stages of Alzheimer's to discuss her situation. "I wish, more than anything, that Kath had never got ill. But second to that, I wish that we – I, my wife and my brother – had been able to talk to her about what was happening. We tried, in various ways over the following years, to have frank discussions. But whenever we hoped she'd understand some new limitation, or accept a new level of care, we had to choose between complicity in a face-saving but ultimately pointless pretence and provoking unreasoning anger... Months later, again pretending she didn't need any help, we explained another young carer as a friend in need of a room. Kath, hardly surprisingly, made her uninvited 'guest' so uncomfortable that she left after two nights." Recognizing, as many doctors are reluctant to do, the moral and philosophical similarities between active and passive euthanasia, he adds that "Withholding medication isn't any more morally courageous than the ancient Greeks leaving unwanted babies on the hillside to die". As for the vital, fundamental question of which self – the pre- or post-Alzheimer one – should have the final say, his position is that "the young Kath isn't here, and the old one is, usually, pretty content". We do not know the precise terms of her living will but it seems that either a brilliant journalist did not make her wishes clear enough (as Polly wrote; "Even those who think carefully about how they definitely don't want to end up find that rational plans, made in good health, usually slip away during a step-by-step medical decline") or that they were clear but her son felt unable to honour them to the letter.

Some friends of mine who knew her well and had often holidayed with her thought that her mental decline began insidiously as much as ten years before it became fully apparent and sent me the following comments. "By a sad irony, the very slowness of her disintegration, and the customary brisk warmth of her manner, probably led those closest to her to underestimate the extent of her perceptual loss as well as her memory loss. This inevitably led to the situations in which she agreed enthusiastically to take on excursions, and even one-off work commitments, which were in reality beyond her competence, with resultant muddle and embarrassment. Her apparent belief, even once she had received a diagnosis of Alzheimer's, that she could continue as before so long as no one in Fleet Street knew about her diagnosis, was a great mistake. As so often in other spheres of life also, it was the attempted cover-up that complicated and exacerbated the problem, tarnishing the very image she was so anxious to project. It also obviously made it very difficult for her family to put suitable arrangements in place for her. Her failure – indeed refusal – to discuss realistically possible future scenarios including death, was surely just part of this general fading of acuity." Like Matthew Parris, "The old, real Kath of years ago had long come to the well–informed opinion that the old and sick should not necessarily be kept going unconditionally, and she was a supporter of assisted dying."

12

The Genetics Of Alzheimer's

To test, or not to test?

A completely different sort of Alzheimer family problem is a very recent one that has been added to the existing pile of Alzheimer problems by well-meaning medical researchers, thanks to the iron law of unintended consequences. In the last decade or so, it has been possible to test for one version of a gene that increases the risk of developing Alzheimer's in the typical over-65 age group. The gene in question deals with a constituent of the brain called Apolipoprotein-E (APOE). You can safely forget everything about it except its initials immediately, but unlike the all-or-nothing gene for Huntington's Disease (if you have the gene, you have the disease; if not, you don't), having the e4 version of the APOE gene simply increases the normal, existing risk that you *might* get Alzheimer's if you live long enough (i.e. about 30% of those who are still alive at 85 and about 50% at 95). Our 46 paired chromosomes have genes from each parent but only a small minority of the individual genes appear to confer an increased risk of major diseases. A gene is said to be 'dominant' if even a single copy on one of the chromosome pairs is enough to cause the disease and the affected person is said to be 'heterozygous' for the abnormality. If two copies of the abnormal gene – one for each of the two chromosomes – are needed before the disease becomes apparent, the genes are said to be 'recessive' and the person possessing them is 'homozygous'.[157] Inevitably, things are less straightforward in real life and if having a particular gene is just one factor in whether or not you get a particular disease – as seems usually to be the case – then having one copy of the gene can increase the risk and having two copies can increase it further. This, too, is different from the Huntington situation where being homozygous – having two Huntington genes, one from each parent – does not alter the severity, course or age of onset.[158] All it does is to condemn all of your offspring to the disease instead of just 50% of them.

APOE status sometimes becomes known from the commercially available genetic profiles that some people obtain for entirely non-medical reasons, such as researching their ancestry. It is also a medical research tool and is sometimes done by clinicians if Alzheimer dementia appears to be unusually common in a particular family but some of those family members may also want to know, even if the doctors don't. It is a general rule of screening programmes that you don't screen routinely for diseases that cannot be treated or prevented, because all you do is make people more anxious but that only applies to large-scale screening. We have seen that most potential Huntington patients reject testing and while one might criticize them for not taking advantage of the new technologies that can prevent their offspring from getting the

---

[157] Some genes on the X and Y chromosomes that determine our sex behave differently but in the current state of knowledge, none of them is relevant to this discussion.

[158] Alonso ME, Yescas P, Rasmussen A, Ochoa A, Macías R, Ruiz I, Suástegui R. Homozygosity in Huntington's disease: new ethical dilemma caused by molecular diagnosis. Clin Genet. 2002 Jun;61(6):437-42.

disease and passing it on in turn, it is surely understandable that many of them prefer to remain ignorant. As an old – if questionable – Russian proverb puts it: "It is good to know the truth but it is better to be happy".

When APOE testing is done by doctors or researchers, it is routine to offer – or even insist on – standard genetic counselling before the tests are done or the results imparted. A large US project called REVEAL (Risk Evaluation and Education for Alzheimer's Disease) studied the consequences of revealing their APOE status to adults with no symptoms of dementia but with a sibling or parent affected by Alzheimer's and concluded that the risks of being made unhappy or worse by bad genetic news were small.[159] However, they excluded anyone diagnosed with depression or anxiety and only three of the 81 informed subjects were homozygous for e4 APOE.

More recently, one of the REVEAL team studied 26 people (20 of them women) who had discovered their APOE status from the same commercial source either accidentally or deliberately but without any counselling or preparation. Although the company provided a 'trigger warning' and a short video to help their clients to understand the results, many of them just clicked on the results straight away. Their immediate reactions varied from the unsurprised or stoic to the horrified but a year later, most of them felt that the information had had a beneficial effect overall.[160] Interestingly, the six men in the group were the least distressed by the news. The title of the paper – "Well, good luck with that" – refers to the rather heartless comment made by a GP to one client who shared

---

[159] Zallen D. Green RC, Roberts JS, Cupples LA, et al. Disclosure of APOE genotype for risk of Alzheimer's disease. N Engl J Med 2009;361:245-254.

[160] Zallen D. "Well, good luck with that": reactions to learning of increased genetic risk for Alzheimer disease. Genetics in Medicine. doi:10.1038/gim.2018.13

the information with him. Most of the 26 made changes in their lifestyle, such as diet and exercise, that they perceived as helpful in reducing the risk of getting Alzheimer's. Whether or not it actually made any real objective difference, the very powerful placebo and non-specific effects of 'doing something' (as opposed to doing nothing) would tend to make them feel better, regardless of the nature of that 'something'. A recent Greek study suggests that a 'Mediterranean Diet', especially fish and unprocessed grains, may (and it is only 'may') confer modest protection. Dementia rates are somewhat lower in Greece than the average but as the authors caution, any benefits of the Mediterranean diet cannot be assumed to extend beyond "traditional Mediterranean populations" with their own particular genetic mix.[161] Still, if one has already spent many years both eating and enjoying a fairly Mediterranean diet, as I have, perhaps one can be forgiven for adding a slight smugness to the pleasures and benefits of the diet itself – at least until new research suggests that perhaps the Mediterranean Diet isn't as beneficial as the early enthusiasts thought. Another allegedly preventive measure – keeping one's mind occupied after retirement on the 'use it or lose it' principle – appears not to work.[162] What that study does indicate, however, is that people with a high IQ are less at risk of Alzheimer's than people with a low IQ, presumably because they have an intellectual (or cognitive) reserve that allows them to lose some brain cells without becoming noticeably impaired, just as fat people presumably survive famines better than thin people.

---

[161] Anastasiou CA, Yannakoulia M, Kosmidis MH, et al. Mediterranean diet and cognitive health: Initial results from the Hellenic Longitudinal Investigation of Ageing and Diet. PLoS One. 2017 Aug 1;12(8):e0182048. doi:10.1371/journal.pone.0182048. eCollection 2017.

[162] Staff Roger T, Hogan Michael J, William Daniel S, Whalley L J. Intellectual engagement and cognitive ability in later life (the "use it or lose it" conjecture): longitudinal, prospective study BMJ 2018; 363 :k4925

US studies have shown some interesting differences between various ethnic groups in their risk of getting Alzheimer's but it is not clear that this relates to differences in APOE. Both Pacific Islander and Native American/Alaskan origins confer a lower risk compared with the white non-Hispanics who are currently the majority population. Black Americans have the highest risk and there is also evidence that education is a protective factor.[163] This could be related to social factors adversely affecting early brain development or educational access but those factors might be equally present in marginalized Amerindian and Inuit communities. As well as higher levels of education, higher levels of conscientiousness also appear to have a protective effect. It may be quite a large effect, the least conscientious 10% having nine times the risk of the top 10%.[164] Since conscientiousness is a personality trait that appears early in life and probably has a significant genetic element, there is probably not much point in trying to become more conscientious when intimations of mortality (and worries about Alzheimer's) begin to trouble us in our middle years.[165]

My own feeling about APOE testing is that in the absence of an effective treatment, it is largely unnecessary because *everybody* should be prepared for the possibility of getting Alzheimer's. Even a test that usefully predicted early-onset dementia would only mean that those at risk should make those preparations

---

[163] Matthews KA, Xu W, Gaglioti AH, et al. Racial and ethnic estimates of Alzheimer's disease and related dementias in the United States (2015–2060) in adults aged ≥65 years. Alzheimers Dement. 2018 Sep 17. pii: S1552–5260(18)33252–7. doi: 10.1016/j.jalz.2018.06.3063.

[164] Wilson RS, Schneider JA, Arnold SE, Bienias JL, Bennett DA. Conscientiousness and the incidence of Alzheimer disease and mild cognitive impairment. Arch Gen Psychiatry. 2007 Oct;64(10):1204–12.

[165] Intriguingly, the study involved "997 older Catholic nuns, priests, and brothers without dementia at enrollment, recruited from more than 40 groups across the United States. At baseline, they completed a standard 12-item measure of conscientiousness".

even earlier than the rest of us. Conversely, people who prefer not to think about it and thus not to prepare for it are not going to get themselves tested at any stage. For this very numerous head-in-the-sand brigade, "Well, good luck with that" is perhaps a more appropriate response. As with almost everything to do with dementia in general and degenerative, Alzheimer-type dementia in particular, what you do about it is largely decided by your personal philosophy, world-view or tastes and your situation. The next chapter shows that people can react very differently to the same situation and it is very difficult to say that one reaction is clearly better than another.

13

Not Everyone Can be a Hero; Not Everyone Wants to be a Hero

Lessons from the Holocaust.

Two additional arguments are sometimes used by opponents of deliverance in dementia and in most other scenarios involving intractable illnesses. One is that miracles (or unexpected recoveries) happen and that one can always hope for one. For the main types of dementia, that is not very persuasive because just as God cannot heal amputees (though science has recently produced some very user-friendly prostheses) it seems that he cannot heal people with Alzheimer's either. The only person who was said to have completely recovered from it was the financier and convicted fraudster Ernest Saunders, who successfully appealed against the length of his prison sentence on the grounds that he had developed an early onset version of Alzheimer's. (He was then in his mid-50s.) Although other expert psychiatric witnesses testified that if he had any psychiatric diagnosis, it was depression – arguably an understandable response to being shamed and imprisoned – he was released after ten months instead of fifteen. His subsequent complete recovery and return to the world of finance (where his previous record of making employees redundant apparently led to his being nicknamed 'Deadly Ernest') has since been the subject of many contemptuous jokes among psychiatrists at the expense of both Saunders and the neurologist who argued that he had early dementia.[166] The lack of promising medicines for Alzheimer's (and of the prospect for imminent 'breakthroughs') has already been discussed.

The other argument is that choosing to die according to one's own timetable rather than the timetable imposed by dementia is both a form of cowardice and sets a bad example to other people, especially to the congenitally or long–term disabled who will allegedly feel under pressure to end their lives (as discussed in Chapter 9). In its more purely religious form, as we have seen, the argument may include the idea that suffering is part of God's plan and that it may also be ennobling. The implication is that we should all aspire to be heroes but apart from any philosophical and theological objections to this line of thinking, not everyone is cut out by temperament or circumstances to be a hero.

In this chapter, I compare the various ways in which people respond to a diagnosis of dementia – from contemplating suicide at one end of the spectrum to deciding to   soldier on or simply ignoring it at the other end – with the ways in which many people confronting a different type of catastrophe had to make equally grim choices at a particular point in 20th century history. The well-documented catastrophe I have in mind is what led to very large numbers of suicides among European Jews facing deportation to concentration or extermination camps and knowing or suspecting what awaited them there. I do not think it is inappropriate, or insulting to the memory of Holocaust victims, to argue that the awful end that so worried Oswald Alving in *Ghosts* bears comparison with the awful end

---

[166] https://www.independent.co.uk/voices/profile-ernest-saunders-out-of-jail-and-back-in-business-1347932.html

– in the ghettoes, the work-camps and, later, in the nakedness of the gas-chambers – that worried so many European Jews.[167] In any case, among the members who attended the annual meetings of the old Voluntary Euthanasia Society, there seemed to be a disproportionate number of European Jews who had settled in Britain as refugees from Nazi persecution. These people, I remember thinking, knew better than most of us the important distinction between *voluntary* euthanasia and the involuntary and malevolent variety – a distinction that often seems to be deliberately blurred by our opponents. 'Euthanasia' – in the context of a terminal or intolerable illness – simply means a freely-chosen pleasant or easy death, as opposed to the various unpleasant ways of dying that would be the alternative. There was nothing either pleasant or freely-chosen about the various Nazi techniques and settings that characterised the 'final solution'.

Most western and central European countries or individual cities under Nazi control continued to record mortality statistics in the early years of WW2 before sheer numbers made it difficult. We therefore have reasonably reliable information about the numbers of those who – knowing that they faced a humiliating and undignified fate that might include extermination, even if that was not Nazi policy until later in the war – decided that they would at least die in a more dignified way. What the figures reveal is by far the highest rates of suicide since reliable records began. In one city towards the end of the war, when what went on at the death camps must have become even more obvious than it might have been when the 'final solution' was initiated in 1941, some 10% of its Jewish inhabitants killed themselves when they realised that deportation was imminent. Since not all attempts at suicide are successful, even when they are deadly

---

[167] An old friend who escaped from Vienna in 1938 aged ten, assured me that the comparison was none of those things.

serious – and especially when the method used involves the uncertainties of an overdose of drugs – it is safe to assume that many attempts failed. It is probably also safe to assume that even more people would have attempted suicide if they had had access to effective methods.

National suicide rates are normally expressed as the annual number of suicides per 100,000 of the country's population (the 'at risk' group) aged more than 10 or 15, since suicide is almost unknown at lower ages. To set the Holocaust rate in perspective, recent European and international rates provide a comparison. The rate in England[168] for men – who commit suicide more often than women – was 15.4/100,000 in 2015. The female rate was 4.9/100,000. The highest male suicide rates in Europe for that year were around 32 and 35/100,000 in Poland and Belarus respectively. With the exception of China, female rates are usually no more than a third or a quarter of the male rates in a given country. The international female record used to be held by Sri Lanka with a rate of around 60/100,000 in the mid–1990s. That has fallen but as a country, Sri Lanka is still among world leaders.[169] Currently, the highest known rates are found among minority tribes or communities within a country, the unfortunate record holders being displaced or culturally uprooted Inuit communities in the far north of Canada and Greenland, but even their rates do not much exceed 150/100,000. Many of their communities are ravaged by alcoholism and other drug abuse as well as deracination on the one hand or the inability to integrate with the majority culture on the other. Sociological studies show that many of these deaths, while often intended, were carried out on impulse

---

[168] Wales, Scotland and N. Ireland have higher rates than England for men.

[169] Guyana seems to hold the current record. Like Sri Lanka and other high-suicide agricultural countries, the easy availability of toxic pesticides is probably an important factor, though widespread awareness of the toxicity of a common local plant was another factor in Sri Lanka.

in states of intoxication and probably would not have occurred had the person been reasonably sober.

In contrast, the European Jews who killed themselves at truly record–breaking rates of *as much as 10,000 per 100,000 of the population at risk* had probably considered their options over periods of days, weeks or even months and most of them were almost certainly stone cold sober when they made the final decision. However, one reason for my using this analogy is to emphasise that the Jews who chose suicide were still in a small minority and that that is also true of people with serious illness who choose deliverance in countries where choices in dying exist (and self-deliverance in countries where it doesn't). If twice or three times as many Jews *might* have chosen suicide if the means had been available as those who actually did so, the overall rate among European Jews as a whole would still probably not have much exceeded 5,000/100,000, i.e. 5% of the population at risk – an enormous rate but still a rather small minority. It may be significant that that figure is very similar to the proportion of people who make living wills in Britain and to the proportion who actually exercise choice in dying in the Benelux countries where the option is well established. It accounted for about 4% of all deaths in the Netherlands in 2016, though many deaths – especially cardiac ones – are relatively sudden and the question of a planned farewell cannot arise.

My other reason for using the Holocaust as an analogy is that it shows a range of human responses and considerations in the face of impending disaster. Perhaps those with young children were reluctant to abandon them, just as living with children was shown to reduce the preference for life-shortening interventions in the dementia survey discussed in Chapter 7. Perhaps older or childless Jews felt that they had less to live for but some desperate Jewish parents even anticipated the actions of Joseph and Magda Goebbels in Hitler's Berlin bunker and killed their children as well as taking their own lives.[170] (In the few months following the *Anschluss* in 1938 when the 'final solution' was four years in the future, some 9000 of Vienna's approximately 200,000 Jews killed themselves.)[171] Different people respond in different ways to the same situations and make different choices; and modern Western society increasingly recognizes, accepts and even praises their right to do so. It also accepts their right to argue their choices and preferences in public as part of that freedom of speech and opinion that characterizes Western society and distinguishes it from despotisms of various kinds and degrees, whether Islamic, Chinese, Russian or Marxist (and – in the past – Christian). In Chapter 8, we saw that after the Christian-inspired censorship of alternative views began to fail following the Reformation, prominent theologians such as John Donne felt increasingly able to question the suicide taboo and to argue the case for self-determination. However, the increase in European suicide that accompanied and may have been related to this open discussion only resulted in an increase from a very small percentage of deaths to a slightly less small proportion. Deliverance not only remains very much a minority taste but is likely to remain one for the foreseeable future, if only because – as studies repeatedly confirm – only a small proportion of people, consisting mainly of well-educated, psychologically robust and open-minded citizens, are in the habit of both contemplating and psychologically preparing for their own deaths. Perhaps that describes you, reader, in which case you may have triumphed over the terrifying idea that, as the playwright Samuel Beckett put it, "Everything that man does

---

[170] Many senior Nazis – and sometimes their families – killed themselves at the end of the war. So did many civilians in the East of Germany as fear of being raped by Soviet soldiers spread. So did two of the 23 German generals facing capture at Stalingrad.

[171] Scheyer M. Asylum: a survivor's flight from Nazi–occupied Vienna through wartime France. London. Little, Brown. 2016, 9.

in his symbolic world is an attempt to deny and overcome his grotesque fate". Or in Dr Samuel Johnson's version – and he was clearly terrified by the prospect – "All of life is but keeping away the thoughts of death".

Given that the large majority of Jews who knew that they were about to be deported did not attempt suicide, and that even in the death camps suicide was evidently notable for its rarity, it cannot be argued that the minority who did choose it – in the camps or before being sent there – had a major influence on the others. In the same way, I do not think that providing choice in dying to people who want to avoid an unpleasant and undignified death from dementia will have much effect on the majority who, as it were, prefer the uncertainty and unpleasantness of a journey in the advanced dementia cattle-truck to the certainty that they will never have to board the train in the first place. It will surely have even less effect on those who simply prefer not to think about the cattle-truck at all. Bear in mind that of potential UK sufferers from Huntington's Disease – the most inheritable and predictable of all the dementias – *fewer than a fifth* even seek the genetic testing for the condition that has been available since 1993.[172] In the Netherlands, around a fifth of Motor Neurone Disease patients chose deliverance between 1994 and 1998 but the figure did not increase and actually fell slightly to 16.8% between 2000 and 2005.[173]

I end this chapter by noting that deliberately and prematurely leaving life remains a minority choice not only for European

---

[172] Baig SS, Strong M, Rosser E, et al. 22 Years of predictive testing for Huntington's disease: the experience of the UK Huntington's Prediction Consortium. European Journal of Human Genetics. 2016;24(10):1396–1402. doi:10.1038/ejhg.2016.36.

[173] Maessen M, Veldink JH, Onwuteaka-Philipsen BD, de Vries JM, Wokke JH, van der Wal G, van den Berg LH. Trends and determinants of end-of-life practices in ALS in the Netherlands. Neurology. 2009 Sep 22;73(12):954–61. doi: 10.1212/WNL.0b013e3181b87983.

Jews facing the gas chambers, Dutch Motor Neurone Disease patients facing slow asphyxiation and Alzheimer patients facing the cerebral and intellectual equivalent of slow asphyxiation but also for modern Existentialist philosophers who maintain, among other things, that life is ultimately futile. One of them, Albert Camus, famously wrote, in *The Myth of Sisyphus*, that "there is only one truly serious philosophical problem, and that is suicide". A few leading Existentialist philosophers did actually commit suicide but they seem to have done so mainly for non-existentialist reasons, including terminal or painful illnesses. All things considered, most of them seem to have found life sufficiently interesting and enjoyable to stay around to watch the show and perhaps make a few suggestions for improving the script or staging. I put myself in that category. Of the intellectual professions, poets seem to have by far the highest suicide rate. Should we therefore discourage poetry?

14

The Really Difficult
Future Debate

Should we accept requests for deliverance in living wills/advance decisions when mental capacity has been lost?

I don't propose that the ideas discussed in this chapter should be added to the current reasons for legalizing MAID in Britain; and when – or if – such laws arrive, I would not expect them to be expanded to include these ideas any time soon. Like My Death, My Decision, I personally will be very satisfied if Britain passes something like a Benelux-style law; or even a Canada-style law, provided that it includes early dementia and very slowly progressive neurological conditions. Not tying 'permission to leave life' to a six-month or even a twelve-month life expectation allows people to obtain deliverance when *they* feel they have suffered enough, rather than when other people tell them they have suffered enough. I want them, in short, to be able to share the reassurance that so many doctors can rejoice in. Merely knowing that we have a guaranteed escape route often makes our sufferings much easier to bear. As Nietzsche wrote: "The thought of suicide is a great comfort and with its help I have got through many a bad night". Hardly 20% of the

British terminal cancer patients who get the 'green light' from one of the Swiss organisations actually take up the offer. For many of the others, it is simply a welcome insurance against palliative care that may be insufficiently palliative, but a law that excludes people like Tony Nicklinson and Omid T would be seriously inhumane. Tony Nicklinson had locked-in syndrome and could have lived for another 30 years if he had not stopped eating when his case was rejected by the courts. Omid T had multiple systems atrophy – a kind of supercharged Parkinsonism. Ironically, he was given less than six months to live in 2015, yet when he finally went to Switzerland in 2018, he looked to me as if he might live for several more years, so slowly was his disease progressing. Despite the major ethical and practical considerations, there seems to be a growing feeling in the West-European/Old-Commonwealth nations that advanced dementia should be added to the list of conditions for which deliverance is a rational and medically acceptable option for those who want it. When a Parliamentary Select Committee on Dying with Dignity offered Quebec citizens the chance to make their views known through an online questionnaire, of the 74% of the 6,558 respondents who agreed with legalising Voluntary Euthanasia in specified situations, 80% selected "adults capable of deciding for themselves" but almost as many – 78% – selected "*people who make the request in advance in anticipation of incapacity*."[174] Significantly, the title of a recent Dutch paper about this debate is: "Would we rather lose our life than our self?"[175]

---

[174] Cited in: Bravo G, Rodrigue C, Arcand M, et al Are informal caregivers of persons with dementia open to extending medical aid in dying to incompetent patients? Findings from a survey conducted in Quebec, Canada. Alzheimer Dis Assoc Disord. 2018 Jul-Sep;32(3):247-254. doi: 10.1097/WAD.0000000000000238

[175] Hertogh CM, de Boer ME, Dröes RM, Eefsting JA. 2007. Would we rather lose our life than our self? Lessons from the Dutch debate on euthanasia for patients with dementia. Am J Bioeth 7(4): 48–56.

The debate about how to manage the increasing numbers of patients with advanced dementia may be bedevilled by that previously mentioned "pervasive failure — by both physicians and the public — to view advanced dementia as a terminal illness" but the debate is already under way and quite vigorous. Canada passed Medical Assistance in Dying (MAID) legislation in 2016 and it permits both medically-assisted suicide and voluntary euthanasia. In Quebec, MAID was legalized in 2015 but the lethal medication must be administered by physicians and medically-assisted suicide is not allowed. However, in both jurisdictions at present, MAID cannot be considered for patients who have lost mental capacity, even if they have made a living will that requests it. As in the Netherlands, increasing experience and acceptance of MAID in the relatively uncontroversial context of terminal or progressive illness has meant that discussion about cautious expansion of the permitted indications is taking place, as already noted. Surveys have begun to explore the attitudes of doctors, nurses, senior citizens and dementia caregivers to extending MAID to patients with advanced or terminal dementia who may have lost mental capacity months or years previously.

A survey in Quebec that questioned family caregivers of people with dementia, contacted through Alzheimer Societies, used "a series of vignettes featuring a person with Alzheimer disease to investigate respondents' attitudes towards MAID.... Two-thirds...found it acceptable to extend MAID to an incompetent patient at an advanced stage of Alzheimer disease who had made a written request while competent, and 91%... found it acceptable at the terminal stage. Self-determination was the most widely endorsed argument in favor of access to MAID for incompetent patients. Findings suggest strong support among informal caregivers for extending MAID to incompetent patients, provided they are terminally-ill and had made a written request before losing capacity".[176]

---

[176] Bravo G, et al. Op Cit.

A similar survey by the same team among 291 Quebec nurses asked whether respondents would agree to MAID for "A 75 years old retired teacher, diagnosed with Alzheimer disease, who writes an advance directive in which she refuses all life–prolonging interventions should she be incompetent and *explicitly requests MAID to be carried out when she can no longer recognize her loved ones."* [my italics] 83.5% of the nurses "agreed with the current legislation that allows physicians to administer aid in dying to competent patients who are at the end of life and suffer unbearably. A similar proportion 83%... were in favor of extending medical aid in dying to incompetent patients who are at the terminal stage of Alzheimer disease, show signs of distress, and have made a written request before losing capacity". Almost as many – just over two-thirds – agreed with "providing continuous deep sedation at this terminal stage of the disease, without artificial nutrition and hydration, at the request of the family, assuming the patient never requested MAID while still competent". However, barely a quarter accepted MAID in advanced dementia "at the request of the family, assuming the patient had made repeated requests orally but never in writing", even though the patient "[had to be] spoon-fed, shows signs of distress and cries a lot. All efforts to control symptoms have failed. The treating physician believes the patient has a few weeks to live". In other words, they agreed with slow euthanasia in late stage dementia when no living will existed but not fast euthanasia.[177]

The researchers then submitted the same clinical examples to some 600 "physicians caring for patients with dementia". The response rate was lower but of the 136 who responded,

---

[177] Bravo G, Rodrigue C, Arcand M. et al Nurses' perspectives on whether medical aid in dying should be accessible to incompetent patients with dementia: findings from a survey conducted in Quebec, Canada. Geriatr Nurs. 2018 Jan 3. pii: S0197–4572(17)30319–1. doi: 10.1016/j. gerinurse.2017.12.002

"In advanced dementia, 45% of physicians supported giving the patient access to MAID with a written request, and 14% without such request. At the terminal stage of dementia, these proportions increased to 71% and 43% respectively, reaching 79% and 52% among family physicians".[178] That is quite close to what the patients in my informal survey and the indigenous respondents to the 2007 SE England survey appeared to want but as we have seen, it is not what most of them are likely to get.

One practical problem with this approach is that although many people for whom religious doctrines are not important clearly want to be euthanatized if they were to become severely demented, it could be difficult to do so transparently, even if it were legal. Might it not be terrifying for a confused old man to be reminded of his previous request and told that the time had now come? That may partly explain its rarity in the Netherlands. "Elderly care physicians and relatives were found to be reluctant to adhere to advance directives for euthanasia. Not being able to engage in meaningful communication played a crucial role in this reluctance."[179] If it were legal, surely the kindest way to honour a written and carefully considered request of that kind would indeed be for Matron, or her modern equivalent, to slip something into a routine cup of tea or glass of wine without any announcement – the solution that appealed to half of the respondents in my informal 1980s survey. That is what happened in a recent case in the Netherlands where, although VE is allowed in early dementia, doctors are less in

[178] Bravo G, Rodrigue C, Arcand M. et al Quebec physicians' perspectives on medical aid in dying for incompetent patients with dementia. Can J Public Health. 2018 Dec;109(5–6):729–739. doi: 10.17269/s41997-018-0115-9.

[179] de Boer ME, Dröes RM, Jonker C, Eefsting JA, Hertogh CM. Advance directives for euthanasia in dementia: how do they affect resident care in Dutch nursing homes? Experiences of physicians and relatives. . 2011 Jun; 59(6):989–96.

favour of VE in advanced dementia (29 – 33% in one survey)[180] than the indigenous respondents to the survey in the UK, where neither is legal. However, there have been a very few cases when doctors have honoured a patient's long-standing request to receive euthanasia when the disease had actually progressed to the stage that they dreaded and particularly wished to avoid. Presumably that is one reason why some avoid it by making an early exit, though it is clear that advanced dementia is also dreaded by many of that large proportion of the general public who do nothing about it.

That recent Dutch case involved a woman who had made such a request but appeared to have changed her mind when she actually got to that stage. She had clearly foreseen the possibility of that change of mind – the product of her degenerating brain – and it was one of the reasons she had repeatedly made it clear that she wanted euthanasia. Her doctors agreed after much discussion but she therefore had to be sedated before the lethal dose and a degree of deception had to be employed (though as we have seen, deception is very common in dementia care). This case – worrying or encouraging, depending on one's point of view – is currently being scrutinized and debated in Dutch society and in medical and legal bodies. Time will tell whether it dents the esteem – consistently among the highest in the world – in which Dutch doctors are held by their patients. And whether it is a precedent or an exception. Another consideration is that if it became widely known that such things happened – as would be inevitable – it might eventually give the numerous patients who are both demented and paranoid some real grist

[180] Bolt EE, Snijdewind MC, Willems DL, van der Heide A, Onwuteaka–Philipsen BD. Can physicians conceive of performing euthanasia in case of psychiatric disease, dementia or being tired of living? J Med Ethics. 2015 Aug;41(8):592–8. doi: 10.1136/medethics-2014-102150. Epub 2015 Feb 18.

for their delusional mills. That would increase both the need for deception and the controversy that the idea undoubtedly generates. (It should be said that bureaucrats are not the only people who have reservations about that sort of thing.)

Several papers about this case have appeared in the prestigious Journal of Medical Ethics.[181, 182, 183] Two of them are viewable in full online. The patient – 'Mrs A' – had made an Advance Euthanasia Directive (AED) that stated: "I want to make use of the legal right to undergo voluntary euthanasia when I am still at all mentally competent and am no longer able to live at home with my husband. I absolutely do not want to be placed in an institution for elderly dementia patients. I want to take a dignified farewell from my precious loved ones... Trusting that at the time when the quality of my life has ended up in the above-described situation, I would like to undergo voluntary euthanasia." Although she may have held these views for many years, she apparently did not record them when she was still in good health and the Directive was made when she was already in the early stages of Alzheimer's, having been diagnosed three years earlier. That may partly explain the ambiguity of some phrases, although it is clear that many people very much want to avoid being 'placed in an institution for elderly dementia patients'. Three years later, she revised the Directive, substituting instructions that "I want to make use of the legal right to undergo euthanasia whenever I think the time is right for this... Trusting that at the time when the quality of my life has

---

[181] Miller DG, Dresser R, Kim SYH Advance euthanasia directives: a controversial case and its ethical implications J Med Ethics 2019;45:84-89

[182] Jongsma KR, Kars MC, van Delden JJM Dementia and advance directives: some empirical and normative concerns J Med Ethics 2019;45:92-94.

[183] Kim SYH, Miller DG, Dresser R Response to:'Dementia and advance directives: some empirical and normative concerns' by Jongsma et al Journal of Medical Ethics 2019;45:95-96

become so poor, I would like for my request for euthanasia to be honoured". The doctor who interpreted these statements as a clear request for euthanasia when the dementia reached the institutional stage (and when Mrs A had actually been institutionalised) did so openly and will defend her decision when the case comes to court. All papers commenting on the case in the Journal of Medical Ethics mention the need for maximum clarity in the writing of Advance Euthanasia Directives and the centrality of the 'then-self versus now-self' problem but they also conclude that the Dutch assisted dying laws, originally designed for and overwhelmingly used by patients whose Mental Capacity is not in doubt, are not really fit for scenarios involving fairly advanced dementia. However, one author argues that an AED could "include in the directive, for example, instructions to administer a sedative (without asking) before proceeding with the euthanasia or to hold the patient down (as family members did with Mrs A). For any such instruction, of course, the appropriate time for implementing the instruction has to be indicated." This might include "when the patient no longer recognises friends and loved ones as the individuals they are or is no longer engaged in even a passive activity like watching TV".[184]

A point I make repeatedly (because it is so important, yet so few people – even highly educated ones – behave as if it were) is that as well as laws permitting assisted dying, an equally desirable legislative change is one that would incentivise the writing and recording of Living Wills/Advance Decisions that clearly spell out in precise and unambiguous detail what an individual wants in the event of moderate and advanced dementia. At some future time, that might involve – as with organ donation after death – an 'opting-out' rather than an

[184] Menzel P. AEDs are problematic, but Mrs A is a misleading case J Med Ethics. 2019, 45:90-91.

'opting-in' system. Bear in mind that organ donation was once looked on as something unusual and exceptional. Gradually, it came to be regarded as praiseworthy but not a matter for any pressure. Now it is regarded as so normal and desirable that consent is assumed unless people specifically refuse. It is another of those 'slippery slopes' but who now would want to reverse the gradient?

15

A Time to be Born and a Time to Die

Why is it right to play God at the beginning of life but wrong at the end of it?

A note on disability terminology.

I showed this chapter to a very prominent disability activist who prefers My Death, My Decision's position to that of Dignity in Dying but wants to remain anonymous. While criticising some aspects of PC thinking, he urged me to change some terms. I accept his contention that the 'social' model of disability is an alternative to the 'medical' or 'tragedy' model and have tried to meet him half-way. So, 'living with disabilities' rather than 'disabled'. However, I cannot agree that it is too 'judgmental' to describe dying from the dementia of Huntington's Disease *and living for many years with its inevitability* as a fate even more 'terrible' than ordinary dementia – which many people do indeed regard as 'terrible'. He prefers me to describe the extra chromosome that underlies Down syndrome as 'different' rather than 'abnormal' but should we therefore describe cancer cells as merely 'different'? He does, however, agree that dementia is different from other disabilities in that (if I understand him correctly) for most of its course and in all cases, patients will be unable to express a coherent view (and eventually any view at all) about how they would like to be regarded by society or managed by their carers. And also, because unlike most early-onset disabilities that persist into adulthood, it will inevitably be fatal within a few years.

Almost everybody accepts that in pregnancy and childbirth, medical skills should be available to make the experience as pleasant and safe as possible and are sometimes essential to prevent disasters to mother, baby or both. I'm not the first writer to argue that medical involvement at the other end of life should be equally acceptable and should not cause fundamental disagreements but in the interval since that comparison was made by – among others – Arthur Koestler, writing in the 1970s, some important changes have taken place in obstetric practice (most of them unanticipated at that time) that involve ethical considerations at least as profound as those that surround Medical Assistance In Dying.

Of the twenty births that I had to attend during my student obstetric training, one resulted in an anencephalic baby and another in a baby with Down syndrome. Anencephaly is the most severe manifestation of a group of congenital (but not hereditary) disorders called Neural Tube Defects (NTDs). At one end of the severity spectrum is spina bifida. It can be so slight that it causes no problems at all but in more severe cases, children are born paraplegic and with no bladder or bowel control. At the most severe end is anencephaly – in which the baby is born without most of its skull and brain. Today, both of those conditions would usually have been detected by the middle trimester of the pregnancy. In many countries – even nominally Catholic ones – the mothers of the affected foetuses would usually have requested abortion, especially for anencephalics, who would not have survived after birth for more than a few days anyway.

The availability of antenatal diagnosis has had dramatic effects on the incidence of both Down syndrome and NTDs. Between 1950 and 2000, the number of children born in Britain with Down syndrome fell from around 2 per 1000 live births to around 1 per 1000, despite a considerable increase in the number of women having babies in their 30s and 40s, which greatly increases the risk of the chromosomal abnormality responsible for the condition. In 2017, it was reported that in Iceland, births of children with Down syndrome had almost entirely disappeared because around 85% of pregnant women request screening and nearly all of them terminate an affected foetus. A CBS report on that situation noted that in the USA, the "estimated termination rate for Down syndrome is 67%... in France it's 77%...and Denmark, 98%".[185]

For NTDs, the changes due to the availability and uptake of antenatal, *in utero* diagnosis were even more stark. In 1968 Britain, there were about 2.4 per 1000 live births with spina bifida and related NTDs. A similar proportion were so severely affected that they were stillborn. The discovery that some cases of spina bifida were linked to low levels of folic acid, and subsequent routine folic acid supplements in pregnancy, reduced the numbers by about half by the end of the 1970s but by the 1980s, abortions for NTDs started to exceed the combined live- and still-birth rate for NTDs, providing (irony alert!) an *in utero* 'final solution' of the spina bifida problem. By 1999, there were only 0.3 per 1000 live births – barely a tenth of the rate 30 years earlier – and 0.1 per 1000 stillbirths; and nearly three times as many abortions for NTDs. A follow-up study 35 years later of 117 babies with spina bifida operated on in Cambridge soon after birth between 1963 and 1971 shows what mothers who decide against testing or termination would have to prepare for. All 117 patients were traced. 54%

---

[185] https://www.cbsnews.com/news/down-syndrome-iceland/

had died, mostly from chronic bladder and kidney infections or kidney failure. Of the 54 survivors, who nearly all had milder forms of the condition, 20 had severe disabilities and needed daily care, in many cases from parents who were by then getting to the age when they might need care themselves. Only 20 were living independently (most of whom could also drive cars) and only 13 were employed.[186] In the case of Down Syndrome – a condition typically (and for many of those affected, correctly) represented as being at the milder end of the learning disability spectrum – parents reported that at an average age of 5 years, 45% of their children needed weekly or daily contact with clinical services.[187] I have already mentioned the use by some carriers of the Huntington gene of the genetic testing of embryos conceived *in vitro* to make sure that their offspring will not share – and pass on – their own terrible fate. The main differences between these particular 'final solutions' and their racist and eugenic predecessors is that the solutions are activated before birth, before the acquisition of full 'personhood', before any possibility of awareness or suffering and mostly before viability.

The first question many of those twenty mothers asked me after their babies emerged – sometimes even before wanting to know the sex of their offspring – was: 'is it all right?', by which I think they often meant: "is it a healthy, 'normal' baby?" Yet – as touched on earlier – while there is some discussion and criticism of pre-natal screening on disability websites, the overwhelming desire of parents not to have children with disabilities has not caused many vocal complaints by the disability lobby. The few

---

[186] Hunt GM, Oakeshott P. Outcome in people with open spina bifida at age 35: prospective community based cohort study. BMJ : British Medical Journal. 2003;326(7403):1365–1366.

[187] Michie M, Allyse M. Gene modification therapies: views of parents of people with Down syndrome. Genetics in Medicine, 2018, doi. org/10.1038/s41436–018–0077–6

published surveys, mostly involving the parents of offspring with Down Syndrome (though not – significantly – the offspring themselves) reveal little opposition to screening but a range of experiences of rearing and caring for them. One participant "called the authors out of concern that the responses to the survey might be too positive because, in her words, it is 'taboo' in the DS community to say anything negative about life with a child with DS".[188] In a long and angry essay describing her debate with the Princeton ethicist Peter Singer, the prominent US disability rights lawyer and 'Not Dead Yet' activist Harriet McBryde Johnson – who relied on a wheelchair because of severe neuromuscular disease – did not even mention (let alone criticise) ante-natal testing.[189]

In my limited experience, the facilities provided by the NHS and social services for people living with severe disabilities are of high quality. In the course of doing Capacity reports for patients who want to end their lives in Switzerland, I visited a few such people and was pleasantly surprised by the resources made available to them and the levels of medical and community support – levels unimaginable when I qualified. Furthermore, although in the late 1970s there was some subdued debate about the management of children born with severe spina bifida (one DHSS leaflet actually suggesting that they could be generously sedated so that they would not want feeding)[190] the views of the preservation-at-all-costs lobby gradually disappeared from medical journals. I even recall (though I cannot find the reference) a letter in the British Medical Journal from a

---

[188] Hippman C, Inglis A, Austin J. What is a "balanced" description? Insight from parents of individuals with Down syndrome. J Genet Couns. 2012 February ; 21(1): 35–44. doi:10.1007/s10897–011–9417–2.

[189] https://www.nytimes.com/2003/02/16/magazine/unspeakable-conversations.html

[190] Brewer C. Life with spina bifida. BMJ. 1977;2:1670

teenaged boy with spina bifida who said that it would be better if the birth of people like him could be prevented. On the other hand, the fact that most children who have lived with disabilities from birth or childhood get used to their disabilities, adapt to them, often mix with similar people and usually spend none of their childhood years wishing they were dead probably means that few of them will change their minds when they are old enough to learn that some people, especially those whose disabilities occur much later in life, find it impossible to adapt and take a different view.

The widespread acceptance of abortion for what are very widely regarded (whatever the disability lobby may say) as 'imperfect' foetuses should theoretically be much more worrying, threatening and stigmatizing to adults living with disabilities than the possibility that some of those adults might decide to invoke laws permitting deliverance from what they regard as intolerable afflictions. However, that is only one of the developments in the mechanics of childbirth and in the manipulation and selection of genes and embryos that have taken place in my professional lifetime. All of them aim to interfere with Nature by way of ameliorating or abolishing natural, God-given diseases and disabilities (or troublesome differences requiring major inputs from family and State) and the hazards of natural, doctor-free childbirth. In the 1960s, childbearing was still a painful business for many British women even in hospital. Anaesthesia was primitive, epidurals were rare, and we were taught that if we did an episiotomy (cutting into the tissues at the mouth of the birth canal to avoid tearing) women wouldn't notice the extra pain if we did it during a uterine contraction. By the 1980s, epidurals were routine. Then Caesarean Section, which had once been restricted to obstetric emergencies, or to women with a history or likelihood of difficult or obstructed labour, began to be increasingly requested by women themselves, as well as by obstetricians worried about being sued if a natural birth looked like being even slightly difficult and might produce an expensively brain-damaged baby. Some of the women were caricatured as 'too posh to push'. Others just wanted to be asleep until the whole messy process was over. Others still, especially in Latin America, requested Caesareans because their husbands – to put it bluntly – preferred tight vaginas to slack ones.

Genetic testing and embryo selection for parents carrying genes for inheritable diseases meant that embryos that would previously have developed into babies with conditions that would blight their development and often kill them in childhood ('differences' is surely a particularly inappropriate euphemism for this category) were discarded in favour of embryos that would develop into healthy children with normal life expectation. Long before these developments, birth control in various forms allowed women to have some control over the number of pregnancies they had to go through. That is one reason why the maternal death rate steadily declined, so that death in childbirth – once common – became very rare in developed countries.

These developments did not go unopposed and in the West, nearly all the opposition came from monotheistic religions. From the use of anaesthesia in childbirth to the provision of contraception – at first only to married women; from the decriminalization of abortion (which abolished unsafe backstreet operations almost overnight) to embryo research aimed at understanding and defeating genetic diseases; from in vitro fertilization to surrogate wombs for the infertile – the churches have either been against them or have dragged their feet before reluctantly agreeing.[191]

---

[191] "It is no longer argued that to assuage the sorrows of childbirth is flying in the face of Providence." Dr Edward W Murphy. BMJ (Association Med J) 1853, 3.1. 780

In contrast, many people – including many doctors – feel that the degree of suffering at the other end of life, and the lack of ethical and medical developments to deal with it, is now much worse for many patients than it used to be. Medicine now enables many more people to reach old age while still enjoying life and taking part in vigorous activities, even into their nineties but it has also produced unprecedented numbers of old people with several chronic and progressive illnesses, for whom death is a happy release from physical and mental pain, often aggravated by loneliness and unrelieved by any continuing ability to enjoy food, music or simpler pleasures. Dementia may shield its victims from an awareness of how much they have lost but that is hardly a recommendation. The extent, intensity and variety of inappropriate treatment that I have described and criticized exemplifies a society (and often its individual members) that, in the words of the widely admired surgeon-writer, Atul Gawande, "faces the final phase of the human life cycle by trying not to think about it".[192]

Few problems of our time are more difficult to contemplate, let alone to solve. Not all problems have a solution and this may be one of them. A long and thoughtful online paper by a US academic lawyer[193] takes that view, though I think that observing his mother's somewhat atypical dementia may have given him a rose-tinted view of the subjective dementia experience and of what can be done in the more advanced stages. The temptation to ignore it is understandable and politicians are reluctant – even frightened – to debate it but there are two basic choices that can be made. Society – and its individual members – can do nothing or it can do something.

---

[192] Gawande A. Being Mortal: illness, medicine and what matters in the end. London, Profile/Wellcome. 2014, 77.

[193] Mitchell JB. Physician-assisted suicide and dementia: the impossibility of a workable regulatory regime. Oreg. Law. Rev. 2010, 1085–1138.

PART 2

RESPONSES TO DEMENTIA:

Doing nothing or doing something.

16
Doing Nothing

1. Individuals

Individuals can make choices about how they respond to dementia. So can societies but individuals can do it much more easily. There are therefore two aspects of 'doing nothing': the personal and the political. I'll deal with the personal first.

As an individual, you may actively prefer to do nothing and simply let matters take their course even though – as we have seen – that course is no longer the 'natural' one. It is decided largely by what others, mainly health professionals, believe is the right level of intervention to thwart Nature. It means (even if many of us prefer not to think about it) that your personality will gradually be replaced by a different personality, which may initially retain some traces of the old one but will eventually cut you off from all human contact and all human pleasure. If you are a member of the home-owning classes, it may use up tens or even hundreds of thousands of pounds that you had intended to leave to your family or to various good causes that were matters of importance to you when you had a mind that could still consider them. Your family may continue to visit you when you can no longer be looked after in your own home but eventually you will no longer recognize them when they do so. You may, if you are in a lucky minority, appear happy or at least not unhappy but you will not be able to share with them the nature of your happiness. Even if you appear indifferent to your condition, that – and the sight of your shrinking and enfeebled body – is distressing enough but your behaviour may cause them additional anguish if you are troubled by pain in your degenerating joints or by frightening delusions and hallucinations that originate in your degenerating brain.

Married women with dementia are likely to have outlived their husbands. If no spouse is capable of the caring role, most families can no longer rely on assistance from unattached daughters who feel it their duty to leave any job they may have and devote their whole lives to the care of demented or merely infirm parents. If the daughters are unattached by choice and have no children of their own to think about, it is likely that they value independence and have careers that are both important to their identities and vital to that independence. The return of the spinster is a very unlikely scenario.

2. Society

In most countries, society – or at any rate, its elected representatives – routinely prefers to do nothing about the steady increase in the number of patients in the advanced stages of dementia. Even though most British citizens do not want to be kept alive with severe dementia, that is what generally happens to them. The cost is – to put it very mildly – considerable. Writing in the Spectator after Prime Minister Theresa May suddenly abandoned her proposed 'dementia tax', Matthew Parris argued that although he did not want to sound brutal, "..the truth is brutal. Where the state is largely or wholly responsible for the care and cost of an elderly person's dementia, no individual has an overwhelming interest in their timely passing. If the state pays for care — often for a decade or more — and upon death the surviving family inherit a legacy that is undiminished by the huge cost of that care, what is it to them that the life has been unnaturally prolonged?"[194]

After noting that until recently, the social and individual burden of caring for "those whose advanced senility means they can bring neither happiness nor usefulness, even to themselves" – and I stress that those are Parris's words, not mine – was limited by the fact that few of them reached that stage, he continued: "That is no longer the case. We have conquered nature at least to the degree that we can prolong life for decades — even if it is not an active, wholly sentient life. The burden this is placing on our economy, on family life, on state spending, and on our health service, is growing fast and relentlessly".

"Nobody", Parris continues, "wants to think about, let alone decide, how long someone they have loved should live when their life has become meaningless. When the cost of life falls upon the general taxpayer, why argue against life? When I am old, and if I then suffer from dementia, it would be painful (I hope) for my (younger) partner to put into train anything that allowed, or helped, my life to end. The easiest thing for him to do will be to put me in a nursing home, visit me dutifully occasionally, and leave the taxpayer to pay the bill — with all my estate headed safely his way when I go. If a tough and harrowing decision can be avoided by sending the bill to the Chancellor of the Exchequer, I'm afraid that's where the bill will go." Parris did not suggest that implementing the dementia tax would mean that millions of British citizens would suddenly "declare they no longer believed human life was sacred" but

---

[194] Parris M. A dementia tax would eventually become a euthanasia bonus. Spectator. 27 May 2017

gradually and "probably over generations, the argument for letting or helping people die when their lives had emptied would begin to find more favour."

What Parris describes is true of Norway, where nursing home residents are expected to contribute no more than about two-thirds of their individual pension. It may be true of a few other prosperous countries too but Parris did not spell out the current financial arrangements for the large number of older British residents who, like him, own their houses and have at least a few thousand pounds or even multiples thereof in the bank or in pension funds. If they require nursing-home care (but not actual hospital-type nursing, which many will not need) they will have to pay for most of it and they will be lucky if there is much change out of £800–£1000 per week at current rates. If that exceeds their pension, as it will for the large majority of people, and whatever small benefits the state may provide, they will have to use up their capital (including, at some stage, the value of their house) to cover the difference. Only when their capital is reduced to around £23,000 will the State take full responsibility. However, what Parris describes does apply to the large number of British residents in the main Alzheimer age group who don't own a house and rely largely or exclusively on modest pensions, sometimes topped up with additional social security or disability benefits. They include a proportionately larger number of the sort of less educated and possibly more religious people who are least likely to think about and plan for their deaths and who may also be more attached to the idea that 'everything must be done'. Not many of them may have much more than that minimal £23,000 in capital or property to leave to their children but it will be welcome enough in a relatively poor family. 'Putting them in a nursing home, visiting them dutifully occasionally, and leaving the taxpayer to pay the bill' is a pretty accurate description for that large part of British society.

If individual patients and family members find that thinking and deciding about these absolutely fundamental issues (and they really don't come more fundamental) is painful, drawn-out and difficult, society – and its representatives – is not going to find it any easier. In Britain, doing nothing looks likely to remain society's default position for many years.

17

Doing Something

1. Individuals.

Dementia sufferers who prefer an early exit to living with steadily diminishing awareness and dignity and – in many cases – steadily increasing distress until they die need to make the necessary arrangements well before they lose mental capacity; and therefore while they may still have at least a few months of life that might bring them and their social and family circle some pleasures to set against their declining abilities and shrinking horizons. That is true whether they seek the Swiss option or plan a DIY approach. It is also true, at the moment, for most citizens of the Benelux countries and Switzerland, where deliverance is possible in early dementia but only with great difficulty (and not at all in Switzerland) when dementia is more advanced. The desirability of going a bit too early rather than leaving it until too late is similar to the dilemma facing patients in Britain or elsewhere with progressive neurological disorders like motor neurone disease who must generally to go to Switzerland before their loss of mobility or the need for assisted breathing makes travel too difficult or too expensive. If the law is changed in Britain, such neurological patients should be able to delay their planned deaths by weeks or months and then die at home, because travelling to Switzerland will be unnecessary. However, for Alzheimer patients, it is not loss of mobility that may determine the timing but loss of mental capacity and that is what usually matters whichever country they live in or travel to.

Forgive me for again repeating that the most important 'something' that people need to do is to accept the inevitability of their own death – and the possibility that it might involve dementia – while they are still relatively young and in good health; to think carefully and at leisure about how they would want serious illnesses and terminal states – including dementia – to be managed; and to make sure that there is a written record of their wishes. Ideally, it should be reviewed from time to time. If, many years later, they request deliverance when they develop Alzheimer's, documents confirming a consistent preference for deliverance will be very persuasive evidence that the request arises from a careful consideration of the options and a consistent existential position. It is also a powerful antidote to the kind of clinician who insists that you are just having a sort of bad hair day – a mere reaction to the news of your diagnosis and prognosis that will pass before long. In these situations, clinicians of this kind are apt to label you as 'depressed' and urge you to take antidepressants. The idea that 'depression' (aka unhappiness) might be a perfectly normal, understandable and appropriate response to the prospect of dementia is one that they are often reluctant to accept or even discuss.

If persisting or increasing awareness of memory problems and/or comments from family and friends eventually make you wonder whether you might be developing dementia, it is important to see your GP with a view to getting assessed at a memory clinic or by a dementia specialist – NHS or private according to taste and pocket, though in my experience, the NHS clinics generally give an exemplary service, at least at the technical and diagnostic level. This may provide the good news that there is no sign of dementia but it also provides some baseline test results. If they show that you do have early dementia, or if you develop dementia later, those baseline tests may be very useful for calculating the likely rate of progression. A slowly progressive dementia may give you two or three years to think, plan and prepare. Rapid progression, obviously, may reduce that window of opportunity to months.

At the time of writing, both Dignitas and LifeCircle will, in principle, accept patients with early dementia who retain mental capacity. It is possible that some Belgian doctors will also accept UK residents if they are able to get to know and monitor a patient for several months and thus develop an ordinary professional relationship in parallel with the treatment team at home and the same possibility may now exist in The Netherlands, though neither country is keen to encourage 'deliverance tourism'. Most NHS GPs and specialists are willing to continue treatment as usual even when they know that a patient is planning deliverance. (If they decline, you should complain very strongly.) Details of the sort of medical reports that the Swiss organisations need, and the tactics that may sometimes be necessary to obtain them are given in Chapter 19.

For physical illnesses that do not impair mental capacity, the Swiss organisations are usually satisfied with a medical summary that is no more than three months old, since capacity is not usually an issue. For dementia, however – and for obvious reasons – the most recent mental capacity assessment must be no more than 21–30 days old when patients make their final journey to Switzerland. That is partly because the Swiss want to avoid a situation where you are given a date but cannot satisfy the Swiss doctor who, before writing the lethal prescription, must make a final assessment that you still have capacity, and partly to protect themselves.

Depending on the rate of progression and the particular type of dementia, you may need to have further assessments at appropriate intervals while you make plans, make a formal application, and find an independent psychiatrist – if necessary – to confirm mental capacity for the application and the final 30-day period. If dementia is the result of, or co-exists with, a more generalized neurological condition such as Parkinson's Disease, you may also have to arrange special transport. If you are very immobile, it may be cheaper and certainly simpler for you and those who will accompany you to hire a small plane (just under £5000 for four people, according to one quote) rather than a private ambulance. It may also be not vastly more expensive than the cost of one or more overnight stays in adequately equipped hotels during a long journey by road in a family car. At the time of writing, nobody in Britain has been charged with any offence – let alone convicted of one – for accompanying a friend or family member to Switzerland. Neither has anybody been charged after assisting someone with making an application, which is often necessary when patients are prevented by conditions such as motor neurone disease or visual impairment from writing, signing or typing it themselves.

2. Society

Matthew Parris, a former Conservative MP, is not widely regarded as a wild-eyed revolutionary and there was no eruption of national outrage following his article. Let us look at a few specific practical policies and decisions that his article implies but does not spell out. There are, indeed, several things that British society can do right now without requiring any new legislation, or the long and bitter debates that any legislative proposals – successful or not – inevitably provoke. Much the most important is for the government and the NHS to encourage everybody, as the churches once regularly did, to think carefully about death and to record their wishes about how they would want to be treated in the event of becoming severely (or even moderately) demented. Standard living wills (or Advance Decisions) do not always make this sufficiently clear but the two important court rulings mentioned earlier clearly mean that hospitals and nursing homes have a legal duty to observe instructions in a living will to avoid assisted feeding and that in the absence of a living will, they have a right to withdraw assisted feeding (or not to start it) if both the family and the physician in charge agree that it is inappropriate. I expand on that idea in the final chapter.

Since people whose living wills clearly insisted on this duty would usually be saving the NHS and the taxpayer tens of thousands of pounds – and sometimes hundreds of thousands – they could be rewarded with a modest increase in their state pension, or a decrease in estate duties. To minimize needless distress for both the patient and the family, it should be accepted by both the NHS and the General Medical Council that if feeding and fluids are withdrawn, generous sedation must be routine between withdrawal and death, as it always is when they are withdrawn in the case of babies with severe brain damage.

There would also, eventually, need to be a parallel debate about Society's attitude to the minority of people who, as discussed in Chapters 8 and 20 want 'everything' to be done – and who expect the State or the NHS to pay for it – even in advanced dementia when the patient has no awareness of that 'everything' and, more importantly, never will have. A few such cases end up very expensively in court when a hospital challenges a family's persistent demands for futile treatment. There must be many more in which futile care is provided for many days or weeks before the families accept that it is, indeed, futile. One obvious solution to this cultural and religious divide (and it is definitely cultural and religious, not racial or 'ethnic') would be to encourage the sects or religions to which nearly all of this minority adhere to fund that futile treatment from tax-deductible donations from within their congregations (both here and in other countries) perhaps with the larger and richer sects subsidising the smaller and poorer ones in the best traditions of mutual assistance, charity and alms-giving. The State or the NHS might provide the architectural infrastructure for these sanatoriums (perhaps 'thanatoriums'[195] would be a better term) but not the staff, the drugs or the equipment and any admission to an acute NHS hospital, with a very few exceptions, would have to be paid for. Matthew Parris would presumably not dismiss this suggestion. The hospitals and nursing homes in which this therapeutic maximalism held sway would be similar, in some respects, to the hospitals that were set up in Britain to cater for particular minorities or religious groups and that still exist in other countries. There were, for example, German, Italian and Jewish hospitals in London that were incorporated into the NHS at its inception and only disappeared fairly recently. The excellent private Catholic hospital, mentioned earlier, to which I used to admit my alcoholic patients would never have admitted them if I had been a gynaecologist and wanted to carry out abortions. In the US, many hospitals proudly describe themselves as Catholic or Lutheran.

---

[195] From the Greek. Thanatos = death.

18

Doing it Yourself

The alternative – self-deliverance – would be unnecessary if assisted suicide or voluntary euthanasia were legal. While some doctors might prefer to enjoy a final exercise of their independence and clinical skills by doing everything themselves, I think that for most patients, 'unofficial', Do-it-Yourself deliverance would disappear in the same way (and for the same reasons) that DIY and 'back–street' abortions stopped happening in Britain within months of the decriminalization of abortion and the consequent availability of safe and legal medical and surgical procedures. However, recent research from Belgium indicates that a small but significant proportion of suicides in the elderly occur in people whose quality of life has been severely reduced by chronic illnesses. Suicide accounts for about 1% of deaths in Belgium. A study that linked suicides to the types of medication taken in the year before their death,[196] and therefore gave a good indication of the types of illness from which they were suffering when they died, found that "About 0.2% of all deaths is from suicides

---

[196] Cohen J. "Overlap" between suicide and physician aid-in-dying. Paper presented at ICEL3, Ghent March 2019.

with a certain 'overlap'" with MAID. They happen "slightly more often in institutional settings and by older persons" and more often involve poisoning and firearms, although hanging is still the most frequent method. Most of the 'overlap' suicides had more than one illness. Some had dementia but the single largest category was severe lung disease, which often gives a very poor quality of life and is difficult to palliate. Since MAID is legal in Belgium, it may be that some of these patients could not easily access it for some reason, including living in institutions that disapprove of MAID. Others may represent desperate patients with conditions like vascular dementia that impaired their decision-making abilities. Others still may simply have been reluctant to share their feelings with anyone else, including doctors. My guess, though, is that many of the 'overlap' killed themselves – as most younger and physically healthier suicides do – rather impulsively, without planning or discussion, not primarily because of their illnesses, sometimes after drinking too much, and without a proper consideration of alternatives.

While – to repeat – this book will not provide any specific advice on the techniques of self-deliverance, I am hardly telling readers anything they don't already know if I note that the internet is informative on this matter as on so many others. Several organisations openly run seminars on self-deliverance – at least two of them in Britain – that have not led to police investigations. One seminar was the subject of an approving and rather light-hearted article in the Spectator. ("It is a sunny Saturday afternoon in Covent Garden and we are all learning how to kill ourselves... The woman next to me is 72; she has been watching Prunella Scales in Great Canal Journeys on television and is worried about dementia, which she points out 'can last a very long time'. She has been a member of Exit for three years but this is the first workshop she has attended. She doesn't want to kill herself immediately, but thinks it is a good idea to have 'something in the store cupboard.'")[197]

The self-deliverance movement has two slightly different but co-existing wings. One began out of frustration with the repeated failures of reform attempts, despite considerable public support for the legalization of deliverance. It saw self-deliverance as a temporary expedient, pending legalisation. The other regarded medical involvement as unnecessary and inappropriate in what is essentially a matter of personal freedom and autonomy. Since necessity is a great teacher, both wings have studied, developed and published techniques that do not require stupefying drugs (which can often only be legally obtained through doctors) and do not involve violent, painful or disfiguring methods (such as guns, pesticides, razors, railways or cliffs). After self-deliverance, the idea is to be dead but not distressing to look at.[198] All the techniques require a certain amount of planning and are thus very unlikely to be used in impulsive suicide attempts. The substances they use are not difficult to obtain and are both legal and virtually impossible to outlaw, but you cannot necessarily just walk into any high street chemist or hardware store and buy them – as you can easily do for a rope, or the over-the-counter analgesics that still cause several hundred suicidal deaths annually. (Paracetamol, still used in many suicidal overdoses, is actually a very unsuitable drug, as is aspirin. Neither drug leads to rapid unconsciousness, which is what many impulsive overdose-takers want, even if they are not really suicidal. Indeed, paracetamol does not lead to unconsciousness at all unless it causes liver failure and that only happens several days later in a minority of people who are genetically susceptible. Even then, it is often

---

[197] Berens J. 'Dr Death' and his £50 suicide workshops. Spectator. 8 July 2017.

[198] As Dorothy Parker put it in 'Resumé: 'Razors pain you/Rivers are damp….'

treatable in developed countries with medication or, if that fails, liver transplantation.)

I think I inaugurated the first, frustration-motivated self-deliverance wing after I was invited to join the committee of the Voluntary Euthanasia Society in 1978. Asked for my thoughts, I said that I would be pleasantly surprised if we managed to get British law changed in my lifetime. (I was 37 then and at 78, it remains likely that I will need to exceed the average longevity for my social class and gender if I want to enjoy that surprise.) I proposed that we consider publishing a booklet, restricted to people who had been members of the society for at least three months, telling them how to end their lives themselves if they felt that there was no acceptable alternative. All doctors, I pointed out, had this knowledge and it was a great comfort, so what could be wrong with sharing it with our patients?

This idea was well-received by most of the committee. When it was announced that the proposed booklet would be discussed at the next Annual General Meeting – normally a sleepy and poorly attended affair – there was great excitement. Unprecedented numbers (about 250) attended and for the first time, TV cameras filmed the AGM, concentrating entirely on the voting for a motion to proceed with the idea. It was carried by a large majority. During the next few months, the membership, which had never been more than about 2,500, rose to around 10,000. I wrote most of the proposed booklet myself, assisted by a VES member who was a pharmacologist. The committee added a few general and cautionary paragraphs and the writer Arthur Koestler, one of our several distinguished vice–presidents, wrote the preface.

I have described elsewhere[199] how our Scottish members helped us to overcome some delays caused by legal anxieties

---

[199] Brewer C. The story so far: from King George V to Dignitas. In: C. Brewer and M. Irwin (Eds) I'll See Myself Out, Thank You. The arguments for rational suicide. Skyscraper. 2015

about publishing it in England. Scotland has a separate legal system, in which suicide had never been a crime and therefore there was no specific offence of aiding or abetting it equivalent to the English one. The Scottish branch of the VES declared independence and with much very willing assistance from us, they were able to publish their own booklet – 'How to die with dignity' – just in time for our next AGM in 1980. It was the first such guide in the world but not the last.

My fellow committee member Mary-Rose Barrington suggested using the term 'self-deliverance' instead of 'euthanasia', which had acquired some undesirable connotations since the Nazi regime's decidedly involuntary programmes. It was adopted by the Scots in their publication and we called our own booklet, which came out a few months later, the 'Guide to Self-Deliverance' – which is why I use the term 'deliverance' here. It also had more positive connotations than 'suicide', and as we noted in the Guide, it is "not a euphemism....There is nothing soft-edged about 'self-deliverance': its overtones are as precisely delimited as those of the more familiar 'suicide.' It implies that the person dies by his or her own hand, with a peaceful mind and for reasons that those closest will endorse. They will know that they were not intended to feel guilt or grief, but rather to share sympathetically in a final display of courage and good sense." We also quoted from the Stoic philosopher Epictetus and the 17th century poet and divine John Donne. ('The keys of my prison are in mine own hands')

For self-deliverance from dementia, it is just as important to be sure of the diagnosis and to try to anticipate the rate of progression. Obviously, it is not essential to obtain your medical records but it is a good idea, partly because if any family member or friend is questioned subsequently by the police, evidence that there was no doubt about the diagnosis might be helpful to them. The main disadvantage of self-deliverance in Britain is that both parties may be more hesitant about the act taking place in the presence of others. The death would have to be reported and there would inevitably be both police involvement and an inquest. There is probably more likelihood of friends or family members being charged than if they had been present at a death in Switzerland, and some possibility of a conviction, though anything more than a conditional discharge or a suspended sentence is probably very unlikely. One way of minimizing the risk of prosecution without foregoing human contact and support at the very end might be a modified version of what Canadian art lecturer Glenn Scott did when he decided to deliver himself from advanced motor neurone disease after his doctors confirmed that it would lead to progressive loss of muscular power, with a slow, distressing and remorseless descent into respiratory failure before death, if pneumonia did not accelerate the process. Glenn was a friend of the well-known actor Miriam Margolyes, who contacted my publisher Karl Sabbagh, a professional documentary maker, about Glenn's plans. Karl made a documentary about it[200], partly because Glenn also wanted his planned death to be used to influence lawmakers. Since Canada has now legalised both doctor-administered and patient-administered MAID, he may well have been part of the reason it did so.

He sold his house, cashed in his life insurance and used the proceeds for a final cultural Grand Tour of Europe with a paid minder, eating, drinking and being as merry as his deteriorating condition would allow. His final destination would be Rome, a city he had filmed, lectured about, explored and come to love, and where he wanted to die – by his own hand. This was the crux of the story he wanted to tell: that he had to end his own life earlier than he would like, at a stage when he still had the use of the hands he needed to achieve the deed. It wasn't ideal, since he knew he could probably have had many

[200] https://www.youtube.com/watch?v=9RXQLF9uTL0

further weeks of enjoyment – however limited – if someone else could administer the drugs that would deliver him. "I intend to take my life, but I must be able to do it myself, and I must do it without implicating anyone else. The laws simply do not allow for disabled people to kill themselves."

When he felt the time had come, he planned a final dinner with friends before sending them back to their homes. "After a sufficient amount of time has passed, preferably enough time for my friends to arrive at their destination, then I'll simply film the whole thing so that there will be no doubt that I did it myself. I'm also leaving in front of me all the documentation – my doctor's diagnosis, prognosis, my will, my Italian will which deals with taking care of house-cleaning after the business." That is what he did a couple of days after the dinner. However, if what I have said about the unlikelihood of successful prosecution – or of more than a nominal sentence if it succeeded – is true, there is probably no reason why self-deliverance in early dementia should have to be a solitary process, provided that it is filmed in the same meticulous way. Unlike Glenn, most patients with early dementia will have no difficulty in handling and swallowing lethal substances, or using the more mechanically demanding techniques. To be present as an observer at a rational suicide is not the same as assisting it. If the likely intention to commit suicide in the event of early dementia was made and documented several years before diagnosis, it would be difficult to argue that friends or family had encouraged it. It is also perhaps rather unlikely that a British jury representative of public opinion as revealed by the surveys mentioned earlier would be able to agree on a guilty verdict. That is one reason why the DPP has to authorize any prosecution under the act and why so few have reached the courts. A guilty verdict in a well–documented case might even ignite public disquiet and lead to further demands for a change in the law.

Having said that, the sequence of events recorded on 'Glenn's Last Tape' arguably strengthens the case for doctor-administered rather than self–administered medication, unless the medication is administered intravenously when the patient opens the tap of an infusion that has been set up by a doctor, as happens at LifeCircle in Basel. Although one terminally ill Oregon patient woke up two days after swallowing his supposedly lethal dose of barbiturates, the massive 15g dose of oral pentobarbitone that is used by Dignitas causes unconsciousness in all cases within no more than three minutes. When it was widely used for sleep, the normal dose of pentobarbitone was 100 or 200mg. In the Casualty departments before barbiturates were largely phased out in the 1980s (a medical rather than a governmental initiative) we used to regard any dose over 2000mg (2g) as being potentially fatal without medical intervention and sometimes despite it, though resuscitation techniques have greatly improved since then. However, there appears to have been no repetition of the single Oregon failure and all families I have spoken with who were present at a Swiss death reported that it was rapid and peaceful.[201] Similar levels of satisfaction and acceptance were found in a larger study of Swiss citizens, which also noted that "Assisted suicide in Switzerland belongs predominately to the civil and private sphere and family members do not perceive it as belonging to the medical domain".[202]

This is Karl's description of what the video camera in Glenn's Rome apartment recorded. "After Elvis finishes singing 'Are You Lonesome Tonight?', the radio blares on

[201] Brewer C. Family members' responses to being present at an assisted suicide: a British follow–up study. Presented at the World Federation of Right-to-Die Societies. Amsterdam May 2016.

[202] Gamondi C, Pott M, Preston N, Payne S. Family caregivers' reflections on experiences of assisted suicide in Switzerland: a qualitative interview study. J Pain Sympt Manage. 2018 Apr;55(4):1085–1094. doi: 10.1016/j.jpainsymman.2017.12.482. Epub 2017 Dec 27.

with a rapid-fire Italian news bulletin. Slowly Glenn shifts round in his wheelchair to the table behind and picks up the bottle of blackcurrant juice. He turns back, and tries to pour it into the bowl....He picks up a jar and shakes something from it into the bowl, probably the contents of the capsules....He then picks up a spoon and tries to stir the mixture. He gets sticky blackcurrant juice on his hand and licks his fingers... As I watch this slow motion behaviour I realise that everything in this last film sequence directed by Glenn has a purpose. The banal Italian pop music on the radio is to provide the police with a timeline to show when the event actually occurred. The candle, slowly burning down, is to show that there has been no editing after the event, to remove evidence of an accomplice, for example... We see Glenn pick up a glass of water with a straw and drink from it. Then he looks up for the first time, breathes heavily and shifts in his chair. He looks around the room. He seems to be thinking. The sobbing voice of the Italian singer rises in a crescendo. And then Glen speaks. 'I want to die...' he says, raising his voice above the music. 'I have done this myself. My greatest fear is that it doesn't work. No one else is involved in this so–called crime. I am killing myself.' He pauses, and as if on some weirdly intended cue, the music changes and the Procol Harum song 'A Whiter Shade of Pale' begins.

'I have prepared for this for months,' Glenn goes on. 'I have [motor neurone disease]. There is no cure, there is no treatment. Death was inevitable. I could not dare to live life as a vegetable. I love Roma so much I had to come here. I apologise to the landlords for doing this on their property. All my dear friends, you have made up the meaning in my life. You are very special to me. I love you dearly.'

He then yawns, three times, and his head sinks on his chest. For the next hour or so, Glenn, apparently asleep, takes sporadic breaths. The radio music continues relentlessly, an anonymous, monotonous succession of pop songs. The Rolling Stones sing 'It's all over now' but it isn't quite, as a deeply unconscious Glenn takes his final three breaths. Shortly afterwards, the candle flame flickers and dies." After swallowing the Dignitas medication, it is not uncommon for breathing to continue sporadically for another ten or twenty minutes though rarely, as in Glenn's case, for an hour. Although he would have been deeply unconscious by then, Glenn's occasional stertorous and shuddering breaths would have worried his friends if they had been able to stay with him, unless they were unusually well–informed about physiology and pharmacology. In a few Dignitas cases, it seems that some features of the terminal illness caused delayed absorption of the drug, so that respiration and heartbeat continued for several hours.

'VSED' – Voluntary Stopping of Eating and Drinking - is often suggested as an alternative if MAID is not available and some descriptions from VSED users (while they can still communicate) and from family observers after death suggest that it is not a bad way to go. That may be true for some people, though it needs a lot of determination to decline food and water if one feels hungry or thirsty. If advanced cancer causes a loss of appetite, as it often does, hunger may soon disappear entirely but thirst may persist, even if the mouth is kept moist with sponges. In any case, people with early Alzheimer's are likely to be in reasonable or even good physical health and will take longer to die than someone who is already fragile. The problem is that the more that small amounts of fluid are given to relieve thirst, the longer it takes to die. When dehydration becomes severe, it may cause a delirious state in which the previous VSED decision is forgotten or denied. Of course, if adequate sedation is given at an early stage, the patient will not ask for water, simple oral hygiene will suffice and death will occur peacefully within a few days.

Another problem with VSED affects patients with painful conditions that need treatment with morphine or other strong opiates. If it is done slowly over a week or two, dehydration increases the levels of morphine in the blood, which sometimes leads to a paradoxical loss of effect and an increase in pain

19

Doing it Abroad

European options and the difficulty of getting medical reports.

Most of the British residents who apply for deliverance in Switzerland have conditions such as cancer and motor neurone disease, in which mental capacity is assumed – as British law also assumes – unless there is a good reason to doubt it. For this sort of application, up-to-date medical records are usually adequate and they often include a 'do not resuscitate' request that also implies mental capacity. However, anyone with a past history or current evidence of psychiatric illness will need a psychiatric evaluation to confirm that a request for assisted suicide is not just due to a transient or treatable mood disorder. Even cancer patients with no history of depression who have been prescribed small doses of the antidepressant amitriptyline purely for its modest analgesic effects may need this. It is not sufficiently known that Dignitas devotes much of its time and resources to suicide *prevention*, rather than assistance. Its motto – 'To live well, to die well' – reflects its well-documented desire to make sure that people thinking of ending their lives because of medical conditions have examined all possible and acceptable alternatives.

Naturally, Mental Capacity is not assumed in dementia. As with other conditions, the Swiss organisations need copies of the relevant medical notes confirming the diagnosis and prognosis and that treatable, reversible causes of dementia have been excluded. If an application is accepted, Mental Capacity will need to be re-confirmed no more than 30 days beforehand. It should not be essential for it to be confirmed by a physician, let alone by a psychiatrist. Clinical psychologists who are interested in brain functions – neuropsychologists – are perfectly capable of doing Capacity assessments and they routinely do the psychological tests that are essential – along with brain scans – for confirming a diagnosis of dementia but Swiss law and custom evidently require a medical assessment. Although it adds to the expense, the 30-day assessment could be done by flying to Switzerland to be examined by a Swiss doctor. In any case, the Swiss doctor who prescribes the lethal medicine has to make a final assessment at that time to confirm that the patient still retains Capacity and thus qualifies under Swiss law.

Since both Swiss and Benelux doctors need to see actual copies of your notes – especially the results of brain scans and psychological tests of brain function – it is advisable for patients to request and obtain them before letting any of their UK doctors know about their plans, if they ever do. You have a presumptive right to copies of your medical notes, after paying an appropriate copying fee, and you do not have to give a reason but the right is not absolute and some doctors refuse on the grounds that knowing the full truth may increase or accelerate your desire for deliverance. This means that you have to appeal and while the appeal may be successful, it may take more time than the progression of your dementia allows you. Scottish law is even more unhelpful and there may be no – or very limited – right of appeal against refusal.

Almost all patients who go to Switzerland for deliverance choose to be cremated there, which is included in the total cost.

Bringing a body back to Britain not only adds several thousand pounds to the cost but also means that both an inquest and the involvement of local police and the DPP are inevitable. In contrast, when returning to Britain after accompanying a family member to Switzerland and cremation there, it is not obligatory to report the death to the police, the coroner or the Registrar of Births and Deaths in the administrative area where the patient lived before the final journey. The family of one patient who did report his death were told very quickly by the Registrar that he neither needed nor wanted to become involved. The only agencies that should be informed promptly are the obvious ones: banks and the providers of pensions or annuities. In these respects, deliverance is no different from the death of a British citizen who has retired to Spain (or Switzerland) and dies there. Here are a few case histories (previously published in *I'll See Myself Out, Thank You*) of people with early dementia who went to Switzerland.

HENRY

Henry was in his early eighties and had been a senior figure in a major industry. A long-time supporter of voluntary euthanasia, he had developed early Alzheimer's disease and the busy social life that he and his wife used to enjoy was no longer possible, because he lost the thread of conversations. Retaining enough insight to realise that things would only get steadily worse and that he might soon not have the mental capacity to decide the manner of his death, he joined Dignitas. When I visited him at his home for an assessment, he met me at the door and clearly understood why I had come and what we had to discuss. Testing showed definite short-term memory impairment but he never lost track of the purpose of our conversation, remained clear and consistent in his desire to go to Switzerland and recognised the consequences of this decision. He was not depressed and not even gloomy. In short, he had mental capacity as legally defined. After a very good life, he wanted a good death and his decision clearly stemmed from existential views that he had held for many years. He also told me that he wanted his sizeable estate to go to his family and not to the staff and shareholders of care homes.

CHARLOTTE

Like Henry, Charlotte had Alzheimer's disease and was in some respects more severely affected but her story has some positive features. It shows that Alzheimer patients who are arranging for deliverance when the time seems appropriate can still get pleasure and fulfilment out of life but there were also some important diagnostic issues. Charlotte's dementia was quite slowly progressive and I first saw her four years after the initial diagnosis. By that time, it had reached the point where an alarm system had been installed in her house because she occasionally got confused and wandered the streets. However, she was able to continue living on her own in a small country town, not far from her very supportive family, and had recently been re-elected to the chair of the local Women's Institute, whose members all knew her diagnosis. The tipping point for her would come when she could no longer live in her own home. That point was approaching but she wanted to hang on until it was very near. Charlotte knew more than most patients about the realities of cerebral impairment because when her husband was still in his sixties, he got very severe pneumonia and the resultant lack of oxygen in his blood caused catastrophic brain damage. She had to share in the eventual decision to switch off his life support.

Apart from assessing whether her mental capacity was impaired by the dementia, I was also asked to decide whether or not she was 'psychotic.' That label had been attached to her following a couple of nocturnal episodes where she was not just confused but believed, during one of them, that some local youths had been banging on her front door. True or not (her daughter thought it was most likely a hallucination or the misinterpretation of an innocent noise) that belief developed into a fear that her daughter had been kidnapped and Charlotte went out to look for her. She was examined at home by a locum (i.e. temporary) psychiatrist who had never seen her before and, according to her daughter, stayed for barely ten minutes. He not only gave her a 'psychotic' label but also prescribed an anti-psychotic drug to go with it. This caused unpleasant side-effects, so Charlotte stopped it after a week.

Delusions and hallucinations are certainly common features of psychoses but in Charlotte's case, they didn't last for more than an hour or so. We don't generally think of that kind of short-lived problem as a psychosis, especially if the patient already has a diagnosis of dementia. 'Psychosis' in this context implies a condition lasting for at least some days and often for weeks or months, during which time medication may be indicated. I thought it significant that all these isolated delusional episodes occurred in the middle of the night. Even young and healthy people sometimes wake in a confused state and hear imaginary sounds and it must be a lot easier if the brain is beginning to fail. There are even special names for hallucinations that occur when people are falling asleep (hypnogogic) or waking up (hypnopompic). They can be frightening but don't normally need any treatment. In any case, there were no signs of any psychotic thought processes when Charlotte came to see me. Indeed, it wasn't immediately obvious that she had any cognitive impairment, since she could follow a conversation and correctly recalled a holiday with her daughter two weeks previously. However, more precise tests of memory showed definite impairments, consistent with the very detailed assessment at her local hospital the previous year. She wasn't at all depressed and said 'I want to make the most of everything I can while I can.' Nevertheless, within less than three months, she decided to activate her long–planned journey to Switzerland, where she had a peaceful death in the presence of her close family. Charlotte took the risk of losing her mental capacity before deciding to go to Switzerland but in her case, it paid off. She was a clergyman's daughter. Her religious faith was probably the strongest of all the patients I have seen and she had a firm belief in an afterlife.

Some advice for doctors who are asked for reports.

The significant number of doctors who discreetly use self-deliverance to escape from unpleasant deaths and intolerable conditions – discussed in the first and final chapters – contrasts very sharply with the attitude to deliverance of the profession's disciplinary body in Britain – the General Medical Council (GMC). The most recent guidelines for GMC 'Fitness to Practise' tribunals[203] tell them, among other things that the guidelines "are designed to protect the public and the wider public interest".

"Our guidance is developed through extensive consultation with the profession and the public. It reflects ethical and legal principles, including the rights set out in the European Convention on Human Rights…Where patients raise the issue of assisting suicide, or ask for information that might encourage or assist them in ending their lives, doctors should be prepared to listen and to discuss the reasons for the patient's request but they must not actively encourage or assist the patient as this would be a contravention of the law… For the avoidance of

---

[203] References to Good Medical Practice updated in March 2013 Guidance for the Investigation Committee and case examiners when considering allegations about a doctor's involvement in encouraging or assisting suicide. GMC/FTPDM/1014

doubt, this does not preclude doctors from providing objective advice about the lawful clinical options (such as sedation and other palliative care) which would be available if a patient were to reach a settled decision to kill himself, or agreeing in advance to palliate the pain and discomfort involved should the need for it arise. … Examples of where such encouragement or assistance might arise include, although are not limited to, where a doctor has prescribed medication that was not clinically indicated:

a) after a patient had expressed or implied a wish or intention to commit suicide, or their intention was clear from the circumstances

b) and the medicine would cause death if taken at the prescribed dose or according to the doctor's instructions."

I'm not sure that this advice will really lead to 'the avoidance of doubt' in such situations. For example, a GP who knew that a patient was considering suicide – whether at home or abroad – might be reluctant to prescribe morphine at doses that were perfectly appropriate for pain relief but capable of causing death if a week's supply were taken all at once. Family members looking for someone to blame (especially if they are feeling guilty about their lack of contact with a father or mother or actual neglect) might make a complaint. Even if the complaint is not upheld by the GMC, many doctors dread the inevitable bureaucracy and paperwork that it would involve. The GMC advice continues;

"Doctors' conduct may also raise a question of impaired fitness to practise by (this list is not exhaustive):

a) encouraging a person to commit suicide, for example by suggesting it (whether prompted or unprompted) as a 'treatment' option in dealing with the person's disease or condition

b) providing practical assistance, for example by helping a person who wishes to commit suicide to travel to the place where they will be assisted to do so

c) writing reports knowing, or having reasonable suspicion, that the reports will be used to enable the person to obtain encouragement or assistance in committing suicide."

That last sub-paragraph c) explains why getting any sort of report, whether from a GP, the specialist treating the disease in question or a palliative care physician, becomes very unlikely once Switzerland is mentioned or even hinted at. Interestingly – given the number of doctors who choose self-deliverance – the GMC is more tolerant if a doctor helps a family member. "If the doctor's actions concern a close relative or partner, for example, it is less likely that they would repeat their actions or pose a danger to patient safety. However, such actions may still undermine public confidence in the profession or contravene the proper standards of conduct expected of a doctor." Given that most of the public almost certainly envy doctors their privilege and the particularly high esteem in which Dutch doctors are held by their patients as noted previously, that 'undermining' seems very unlikely.

Allegations that would not normally give rise to a question of impaired fitness to practise include:

"Some actions related to a person's decision to, or ability to, commit suicide are lawful, or will be too distant from the encouragement or assistance to raise a question about a doctor's fitness to practise. These include but are not limited to:

a) providing advice or information limited to the doctor's understanding of the law relating to encouraging or assisting suicide

b) providing access to a patient's records where a subject access request has been made in accordance with the terms of the Data Protection Act 1998

c) providing information or evidence in the context of legal proceedings relating to encouraging or assisting suicide."

This is still more than enough to make most doctors feel very worried about doing anything that might be construed as 'assistance'. Even GPs who know a patient well and are not unsympathetic to the idea of deliverance are generally very reluctant even to discuss the matter. Though there were a few exceptions, repeatedly during the several dozen assessments I have done – the majority of them not involving dementia – I heard about GPs and cancer specialists who absolutely refused to talk (and in some cases, even to listen) to patients facing the gravest crisis and the most serious and irreversible decision of their entire lives. However, while most doctors would never knowingly write the kind of report that would be needed for a journey to Switzerland I know that some NHS GPs and specialists have been willing to do that. Fortunately, I can call on the services of one distinguished but semi-retired NHS psychiatrist if I think a second opinion is needed, as it sometimes is.

The attitude of professional insurers like the Medical Defence Union and the Medical Protection Society, who would have to bear the costs of defending doctors charged by the GMC or the DPP, is also discouraging. They appear to conclude that the DPP might decide against prosecution in a case where a patient had clearly thought long and carefully before deciding; the doctor had tried to dissuade the patient and was motivated purely by compassion; and that any actions of the doctor were only indirect and peripheral to the final outcome.

However, the DPP's most recent guidance implied that doctors involved in the day-to-day care of a patient might be more likely to attract attention than someone like me who is not acting in that capacity. Both the GMC and the defence organisations say that as well as not encouraging any individual assisted suicide, doctors should make it clear that they *discourage* such a course. When I do an assessment, I regard it as both routine and important to make as sure as I can that the diagnosis is not in doubt and that every reasonable treatment option has been considered. Occasionally, I suggest an option that has not been offered, or considered. Rarely do I have any criticism of the way the NHS has handled the diagnosis and treatment up to that point but in one extremely complex current case, I felt it had not done so and I was able to get the patient assessed for admission to a specialist unit which has provided a place on its waiting list. It will, I hope, be able to provide enough improvement to make suicide a less compelling option, provided that the wait is not too long.

During an informal discussion with a senior official from the DPP's department after he had spoken at a Royal Society of Medicine symposium on choices in dying, I put it to him that I could not see how writing a report could, in itself, constitute an offence (as the GMC guidance claims that it would) because some of my reports concluded that the patient did not have sufficient Mental Capacity to choose deliverance, or that not all reasonable treatment options had been exhausted. How, I asked him, could I be prosecuted for writing a report if it came to Conclusion X but not prosecuted if it came to Conclusion Y? A capacity report is simply that. It may say that a patient is able to make decisions about his or her treatment, including decisions not to have further treatment or to discontinue current treatment, or to seek deliverance, but I scrupulously avoid any suggestion that the patient *ought* to seek deliverance and by the time I am asked to see such people, they have already made it very clear over many months or even years that deliverance is what they are interested in, even though – as noted – many cancer patients do not actually go to Switzerland if palliative care proves adequate. He agreed with my view – but as he pointed out, he was not the DPP.

To my knowledge, just as no family member (or TV journalist or cameraman) has ever been prosecuted for accompanying someone to Switzerland for an assisted suicide, no doctor has ever been prosecuted, let alone convicted, for writing a report knowing that it was needed for one of the Swiss organisations. I don't think any doctor has actually had to face the GMC for doing so either. In real clinical life, it is not inevitable that any such report would come to the attention of the GMC because neither they nor the police have jurisdiction over Swiss correspondence or case notes. The NHS doctors who were willing to write reports may have typed them themselves without mentioning anything in the notes. A colleague or a policeman investigating the case might report it to the GMC if it came to light but I do not think the police routinely do that. Even after publicly accompanying several people to Switzerland, my friend and fellow-campaigner Dr Michael Irwin – a former Medical Director of the United Nations – has not been prosecuted, apparently because it is 'not in the public interest' to do so.

As a postscript to this discussion of GMC advice, I should point out that the GMC – like the BMA – has done at least one complete U-turn on a major medico-ethical issue in my professional lifetime and I confidently expect it to do the same with MAID. In what passed for our education in medical ethics when I qualified in 1963, abortion was one of the 'Five As' (along with Adultery, Alcoholism, Addiction and Associating with unqualified midwives) that we were urged not to get involved with if we wanted to avoid trouble with the GMC. At that time, abortion was illegal except for pressing medical reasons but there was a legal grey zone in which it might be ignored – very much like accompanying someone to Dignitas before the DPP was forced to spell out his prosecution policy.

NHS gynaecologists who did abortions for medical or even social indications were often left alone, especially in Scotland where – as with suicide – the law differed slightly from that in England. In Aberdeen during the early 1960s, Professor Sir Dugald Baird would, if requested, openly terminate the pregnancy of any unmarried woman and of any married woman with more than two children but private abortionists doing the same thing were regularly suspended or erased from the Register (and sometimes imprisoned) until the law changed in 1967. Nobody can be forced by the 1967 Act to do abortions or directly refer patients for one if they have a conscientious objection but before many years had passed, the GMC would take action if an objector refused to refer a patient to another doctor who had no such objection. As things stand, the GMC has at least made it clear that doctors who prolong a patient's life contrary to instructions in the living will (as in the case of Miss B mentioned earlier) risk serious professional sanctions.[204]

Since I am no longer on the medical register, like many elderly doctors, I can ignore the GMC. Successive DPPs apparently know that I have written reports for patients considering the Swiss option but I have never been contacted by the DPP's department. The only police officer I ever encountered in connection with a report merely wanted a routine signed confirmation that I had written it. When I asked her if the DPP was interested in my activities or in my reports, she assured me that he was not. Since she was quite a senior officer and the assurance was given several years ago, I assume I would have heard by now if she had been mistaken.

If doctors can, in practice, write such reports with little or no fear of prosecution, then I would like to end this chapter

---

[204] https://ukhumanrightsblog.com/2010/05/20/gmc-to-announce-policy-of-striking-off-doctors-who-prolong-the-lives-of-terminally-ill-patients-against-their-wishes/

with a plea for assistance in the paperwork of deliverance. Until recently, most doctors remained on the medical register (and thus subject to the GMC) and were thus able to continue practising for several years after they retired from the NHS. The cost of staying registered was minimal and it enabled them to help out their old general practice or hospital department when holiday cover was needed, or to see and prescribe for the odd private patient or family member; or because they simply enjoyed their work and didn't want to stop. Today, staying on the register involves mind-numbing amounts of bureaucracy and costs more money than might be earned from helping colleagues out for the odd week or two. This means that the NHS has lost a large and valuable source of experienced doctors (and sometimes of continuity of care) but it must also mean that there are now many recently retired GPs, psychiatrists and other specialists who, like me, can completely ignore the GMC and could therefore share what is likely to become an increasing workload. Provided the doctors writing reports have the appropriate skills and experience, the Swiss are not concerned about their registration status and if any retired doctor reading this would like to help, please get in touch. Because travel may be difficult for terminally ill patients, home visits are often necessary and help from doctors living in parts of the country far from London would be especially welcome.[205] Both practising and retired doctors can also help to shape public and Parliamentary opinion by joining societies like My Death My Decision and their medical counterparts.

---

[205] Home visits are now rare in the NHS but I usually enjoyed them and you can get a lot of useful information that doesn't always emerge in the consulting room. They are still common in private practice. Do you think the Queen sits in Harley Street waiting rooms reading old copies of *Country Life*? Of course not. The members of the Medical Household (who used to have splendidly Ruritanian titles like 'the Queen's aurist' – her ENT specialist – or 'the accoucheur to the Queen' – her obstetrician) go to Her, not vice versa.

20

A Final Word About Doctors and Our Privileged Access to Self-Deliverance

Following the conviction of the medical mass-murderer Harold Shipman, the actions of the government and the GMC led to what many doctors regard as a paranoid and ineffective over-reaction to an extremely unusual case. One result is that it has become more difficult for doctors working in Britain to do what that Henry Marsh was able to do. A common source of self-deliverance medication for GPs used to be the family members who had cared for terminally ill patients in their homes and who often asked the GP who provided palliative care to dispose of any unused opiates and sedatives. Before Shipman, most GPs – wanting to avoid the hassle and paperwork for a controlled-drugs register and a triple-locked, burglar-alarmed drug cabinet – carried a few of these irregularly-acquired ampoules or tablets of morphine and sedatives in their medical bags. They were technically illegal but very useful in emergencies, or for house calls at night. Post-Shipman, GPs who could have given a morphine injection if they happened to be the first responders at a heart attack or an accident now have to call an ambulance instead. For drugs that were in less restricted categories – notably barbiturates – doctors could also write occasional prescriptions for personal or professional use. When I worked in Australia c.1970, GPs had a monthly free allowance of morphine ampoules for emergency use. Many of our generation took advantage of similar opportunities, though doctors – like pharmacists and vets – are better placed to discover and understand the small number of other reliable and painless ways of making an exit without using barbiturates or opiates (or by using substances that do not require a prescription).

I know personally of several doctors who used such drugs for ending their lives to avoid exposing themselves and their families to increasingly distressing symptoms, or the certainty of developing them. Some were distant relations; others I heard about through medical gossip; a few told me directly of their intentions. Although disguising successful self-deliverance might not be easy (or desired) in patients like my friend with early dementia whose other organs were still in good shape, verdicts of suicide were the exception. When cancer was the diagnosis, even if it was not truly terminal, most of these deaths did not even lead to the inquest that would normally be mandatory for a suspected suicide. If death was likely within a few weeks or even a few months and the patient had been seen by a doctor in the previous couple of weeks, a report to the coroner would not normally be necessary. Even if GPs suspected that the death was not due to natural causes, they would probably feel a friendly as well as a professional bond with the patient and would usually want to protect the family, if possible, from the inevitable public airing of their loss. If a body is buried rather than cremated, there is no need to involve a second doctor who might have some suspicions. It is therefore likely that among doctors, more deaths are due to suicide than the mortality statistics indicate. It is certainly true for cancer and one case is particularly interesting for what it tells us about both current UK laws and the ease with which such self-deliverance is concealed.

A few years ago, I got an email from an internationally-known consultant at a major British teaching hospital asking if we could talk. Because I have been prominently involved in both addiction treatment and the Medical Assistance in Dying movement, emails of this kind usually mean that the talk will involve either a problem with alcohol or opiates, or a terminal or progressive illness. This one wasn't about addiction. Nuala had an unusual cancer that was now resistant to treatment and her dying would be more than usually painful, malodorous and miserable. It was also likely that the really unpleasant symptoms would appear well before the six-month limit of life-expectancy for which Dignity in Dying (DiD) campaign (and which My Death, My Decision think is too restrictive and thus inhumane). DiD's proposed legislation would have required either that Nuala must suffer increasing torments for several months before becoming 'eligible' or that one of her doctors would have to commit perjury by deliberately underestimating the length of her likely survival.

She had plenty of lethal medications for the pain her cancer was already causing. What she mainly wanted to talk about was which of the drugs at her disposal would do the job with the fewest unpleasant side effects and the lowest risk of failure, especially as she wanted her immediate family to be with her at the end. We met at her home in the country, where we had a relaxed and quite cheerful discussion over lunch. On the table was enough morphine to kill several of her stockbroker-belt neighbours and a few older boxes of the assorted sleeping tablets that she had haphazardly acquired over a long career but hardly ever used except for intercontinental flights and jet-lag.

A few months later, she emailed me to say that the time to use the drugs was drawing near and thanking me again for my help. Her death was followed by long and glowing obituaries in the medical and national press but none of them mentioned that she had taken her own life. Her GP presumably certified that she died from cancer but I only learned later from another source that the drug she chose for self-deliverance was not one of those spread over our lunch table, or any of the alternatives that she could have fairly easily and legally obtained in Britain. Instead, she bought suitable medication over the Internet. She was happy for me to write about our meeting and the issues it raised, provided that she wasn't identified and after a decent interval. Fortunately, it turned out that we had a mutual acquaintance and after the obituaries, I asked her if she could discreetly find out from Nuala's family whether they had been with her at the end. Despite dropping several hints, she could not get the family to concede that Nuala had died by her own hand, presumably because they were worried that being present when she swallowed the fatal dose would expose them to police attention for assisting a suicide.

Nuala's dignified exit from life contrasted with the very distressing death from metastatic cancer of a woman whose mental capacity and psychiatric status I had assessed a few weeks earlier for her application to Dignitas. She was facing the same sort of messy death that Nuala wanted to avoid but as she was making her final preparations for flying to Zurich, she quite suddenly became too ill to travel and despite apparently competent palliative care at home and in a hospice, her final weeks were marked by incontinence, pain, confusion and great distress – exactly what she had hoped to avoid. Her family had seriously considered risking an attempt to overdose her with her opiates – as many other families must have considered in this situation. Truly, if any dog had been allowed to linger and suffer as she did, its owners would have been prosecuted and possibly jailed.

The issues raised by Nuala's case are extremely important and involve legal as well as ethical, clinical and philosophical considerations. Was I "aiding and abetting" her suicide (the original 1961 wording) or, in the later version, "encouraging and assisting" it, as specifically forbidden after suicide was decriminalised in 1961? (Lord Justice Denning protested during the decriminalization debate in Parliament that it was absurd to make an offence of assisting something that was no longer illegal.) The law even says that I may have committed an offence under this section "whether or not a suicide, or an attempt at suicide, occurs". Apart from the doctors mentioned above who delivered themselves, discreetly and without assistance, from a variety of conditions (not all of them terminal) that made the phrase 'quality of life' a distant mockery for them and their families, I have heard many more doctors discuss with medical friends and colleagues what would be the best drugs and techniques to use if they found themselves in a similar situation. Were all these conversations illegal and should I expect a 5 am knock on my door from the assisted suicide thought-police for taking part in the one I had with Nuala? I hereby formally invite the DPP to consider this account and clarify the matter, one way or another.

Most of those self-delivering doctors had lived fulfilling personal and professional lives and were supported and surrounded at the end by close friends and family. Faced with some of the modes of dying that are the increasingly common alternatives – about half of them in the semi-public surroundings of a medical or surgical ward or, worse, a noisy and crowded A&E department – isn't a planned, rapid and painless drug-induced death actually a rather good way to go? Isn't it how many of our patients would prefer to die? Isn't it how most loving and far from rapacious family members would prefer to see them die? Isn't it how we prefer our cats and dogs to die? And is it right, fair and desirable that in Britain, only doctors and a few other professionals with the necessary knowledge and access to medication can – perfectly legally – have a death like Nuala's without the trouble and expense of travelling to Switzerland before their illness makes travel difficult or impossible?

Rodney Syme is another doctor who rejoices in the fact that he is "particularly privileged, since I have my medication that will allow me to choose when, where, how, and with whom, I will die. I will not have to go to Zurich and seek help from other humane people. As such, I have no fear of death or of dying. I have no fear of a ripe old age simply because I will be able to avoid an 'overripe old age'." He adds: "Of all the medical conditions known to me, I cannot select any that I fear more than Alzheimer's disease" though he notes that it is often accompanied by other life-diminishing organ failures. "Incontinence is a tremendous affront to one's dignity, and can cause serious social isolation. Immobility, muscular weakness and loss of balance may cause falls, limit physical ability, and again lead to social isolation. For some time, as I grow older, I have pondered whether I would prefer to be blind or deaf. Being a lover of music and conversation, I have come down on the side of being blind rather than deaf but I'm not sure I could tolerate a severe degree of either. [Dementia] would be the ultimate insult". Syme, a retired Australian surgeon, notes that many people very definitely do not want to end their lives in nursing homes ("an oxymoron if ever there was one – not in the least like home and very little nursing") which he has described as "...a second prison system. The likenesses are compelling – one usually enters against one's will by someone else's decision, one's life becomes regimented, one's freedom is constrained, one is confined with others one does not choose to live with and with whom one may have nothing in common, and it is a life sentence". Not content with having his own 'get out of jail free' card, Syme has become a deliverance activist.

My fellow-psychiatrist Dr Anthony Daniels – better known as Dr Theodore Dalrymple, one of our most respected medical writers and journalists – is not an enthusiast for changing the law but in the epilogue to a multi-author medical textbook on Rational Suicide in the Elderly,[206] he writes: "[W]hile I like good food and take great pleasure from it, I would not be unduly disturbed if I were told that I could never eat anything again but cheese sandwiches. However, an inability to read or write would, I suspect (though…I cannot be certain) severely sap my desire to live. Everyone is different in what he finds intolerable and what would render his life meaningless. … many people…would not wish to continue to live with a condition [that] would render all forms of pleasure or meaning impossible…". That perfectly describes even fairly advanced dementia. Agonising over legalisation, he adds: "It seems to me obvious that it is sometimes better – kinder, more decent, dignified, compassionate – to bring an end to human suffering than to let it continue. It is difficult, though, to legislate for such matters as kindness and decency, or to lay down precise rules as to when such clemency can, and cannot be exercised".

He is a kind and decent man and might be a good candidate for one of my proposed 'philosophical collectives', to be discussed shortly. On one point, however, I think he is wrong. Arguing that the "possession" of one's life is not the same as having "unlimited sovereignty" over it, he states: "I, and no one else, am the owner of my house; but I may not burn it down". That is not true. If I own my house and the land on which it stands and am the sole occupant (or make suitable arrangements for other occupants if I am not) then provided it is not mortgaged or insured and its destruction would cause no damage to adjacent property, I can do what I like with it. In any case, when I asked him what he would do in an Alzheimer scenario, he replied: "I think I would want to kill myself if I were facing dementia". People who envy doctors

---

[206] Daniels A. *in* Robert E. McCue and Meera Balasubramaniam (Eds) Rational Suicide in the Elderly: Clinical, Ethical, and Sociocultural Aspects. Cham, CH. Springer, 2017. Epilogue 211–8

their privilege when it comes to self-deliverance sometimes add that of course, it would never do if ordinary people had the same access to the means and the knowledge, though they often exempt themselves from 'ordinary' status. It is almost as if they were saying that doctors are rather special people who can be trusted, on the whole, not to use their knowledge and access unwisely or for the wrong reasons. That is how most people used to regard doctors and I think that most people still do. Trust can certainly be abused but that does not mean that nobody should be allowed to trust another person. I know very little about finance and taxation but I have trusted the same firm of accountants with these matters for several decades. They do not impose their views on me but if I am uncertain about some decision, my usual response is: "you know best". As we have seen, that trust is especially attached to Dutch GPs, who carry out a large proportion of the voluntary euthanasia that happens in the Netherlands – much of it in the patients' own homes.

However, in most of the developed world with its increasingly monstrous regiments of bureaucrats, it is almost inconceivable that the sort of individual medical privilege and discretion that Lord Dawson and many of his contemporaries and predecessors took for granted will ever return. Only doctors themselves can take advantage of it – either personally, or for close friends. However, if individual doctors are no longer to be allowed to exercise their discretion, perhaps some sort of medico-philosophical collective might be allowed to do so. Living Wills and Advance Decisions can only take their authors so far. They can request – even beg – doctors to act in certain ways when capacity has been lost but they cannot always *order* them to do so. Neither, it seems, can they free even sympathetic doctors from a tendency to do things that actually prolong and preserve lives whose pre-dementia possessors would not recognize as their own, and had indicated that they would not want prolonged or preserved. Hence all those pointless and very largely unwanted antibiotics, PEG and naso-gastric tubes, drugs to prop up failing hearts, kidneys and lungs and – in the very last unhappy or unheeding weeks of those lives – hospital admissions with a high risk of painful procedures. These include cardio-pulmonary resuscitation (CPR) from enthusiastic but unthinking young doctors. Many of them are just uncertain and frightened of doing the wrong thing but some embody an occasional, rarely-discussed tendency among doctors to view medicine as a spectator sport played to entertain and impress other doctors. For elderly patients, CPR is rarely successful. In a large survey, survival rates to discharge after CPR in hospital were 18.7% for patients between 70 and 79, 15.4% for 80 – 89 and 11.6% for over–90s.[207] Details of their social and functional outcome were "scarce and contradictory" but most patients with moderate dementia who survived would probably emerge even more demented and difficult to manage after further brain damage due to a period of inadequate oxygen supply to the brain. Fractured ribs during CPR are also quite common and unlike other fractures, those affecting the ribs cannot be immobilized with the result that breathing can become very painful.

Instead of these all-too-common scenarios, I suggest that doctors and nurses should form medico-philosophical collectives in each town or compact region, offering a range of end-of-life philosophies, who could take over the management of patients with moderate-to-advanced dementia, subject to a pre-dementia request. As well as encouraging or even bribing everyone to have a living will that specifically dealt

---

[207] van Gijn MS, Frijns D, van de Glind EM, C van Munster B, Hamaker ME. The chance of survival and the functional outcome after in–hospital cardiopulmonary resuscitation in older people: a systematic review. Age Ageing. 2014 Jul;43(4):456–63. doi: 10.1093/ageing/afu035. Epub 2014 Apr 22.

with dementia, people would also be encouraged – when still in good health – to sign up for their chosen collective in the expectation that when their old personalities had died, or were so damaged as to be unrecognizable, the collective would do its best within the prevailing law to make the same sort of end-of-life decisions that the original personality would have wanted. These collectives would be similar to the ethics committees that now exist in many hospitals to help physicians deal with difficult decisions but with one important difference. Namely, that instead of leaving it to whoever happened to be on the ethics committee and therefore the committee's particular mix of views at the relevant time, every member of my proposed collectives would subscribe to a particular set of views that would define it and distinguish it from other collectives. They would not compete but would simply be there for those who wanted them. As with religion – other than the baptism-at-birth variety – everyone would have a choice.

Thus, the minority of people who would want to be kept alive at all costs – literally – even when severe dementia meant that they would never have any possibility of appreciating the effort and expenditure involved and would never even be able to enjoy simple conversations with their families or caregivers, could entrust decisions about their care to a collective whose members had undertaken to embody that view. The collective could also argue the case for paying for that care, either from public funds or from the faith-funded charities that I suggested (in Chapter 17) should be set up for the purpose. Conversely, a collective at the other end of the philosophical spectrum would offer what might well prove the most popular model of dementia care. Namely – and with only a very few truly unavoidable exceptions – nothing but generous palliative pain-relief and terminal sedation when any life-threatening illness struck, as requested in many living wills but often disregarded or 'reinterpreted' in practice. If the law permitted it, the collective could also agree to honour a request not to be fed and watered when patients reached a pre-defined level of dementia – even if they still requested food – and to be heavily sedated instead. (I remind you that that was once the gist of a Department of Health recommendation about new-born babies with severe spina bifida.) Such a request might be valid at present but would certainly have to be tested in court. People who declined – despite every incentive – to make detailed living wills that included a 'dementia directive', or to sign up for a particular collective, would simply take pot luck, as they do at present, unless society decided that they must make a choice.

Alternatively – and it really is the only alternative unless either the passive euthanasia that I have just proposed or active euthanasia become as legal and uncontroversial a procedure, following consistent and documented previous requests, as cremation eventually became – we can just keep on keeping-on, throwing vast amounts of medication and money at people who are long past caring whether they live or die. Who cannot even understand the concept of mortality; whose lives are either empty or full of discomfort, fear and confusion; who, when still in good health and able to contemplate life with advanced dementia, had often made it clear that they would want to spend as little time as possible in that state; and whose horrifying final condition, if we care to think about it, reminds us – as it reminded Osvald Alving and still reminds Henry Marsh, Rodney Syme, Theodore Dalrymple and me – that life is not always wonderful and that not all things in it are bright and beautiful.

APPENDIX 1

If Only Osvald Alving
Could Have Had Penicillin

*Why neurosyphilis is so rare today and no
longer used by playwrights and novelists to
explore sex and madness.*

Fergus was a Northern Irishman in his late 50s who had never previously consulted his GP. After war service in North Africa, he became a foreman and had been in the same job for over twenty years. Married and with three grown children, he had hardly taken a single day off for sickness and had no personal or family history of mental illness. Naturally, his employers thought highly of him but a few days before his admission, this pattern of rock-like reliability began to change. Normally an even-tempered man, he became irritable and moody and he was admitted to hospital after throwing a toolbox through a window at work. By the time I first examined him, he was lying at attention in his hospital bed, right arm at the salute and endlessly reciting his name, rank and army number. (This was at a time when many middle-aged men had seen active service during Word War II or post-war disturbances in the rapidly shrinking British Empire.)

The history and appearance didn't suggest an 'ordinary' psychosis such as mania or schizophrenia. Since there were no obvious recent stresses, that meant that it was probably 'organic', i.e. due to some sort of brain dysfunction. He didn't cooperate well with physical examination but he had a slight fever and his hands were shaky, so we asked for an opinion from the general medical team. The history from his family was largely negative. They said Fergus was a model husband and father as well as a model employee (though families often say that even when it isn't entirely true). Like most people at that time, he hadn't left the country since the war and, like most men over 30, his drug use was limited to smoking and a pint or two of beer. The medical team sent a senior registrar who would soon be a consultant. I had already taken blood and done a lumbar puncture to obtain cerebro-spinal fluid (CSF) but the results had not yet come back. Apart from the tremor, there were other minor abnormalities on neurological examination. Although I had never seen a case, I was worried that the clinical picture was suggestive of neuro-syphilis among other diagnoses, and I felt that we should start treatment with penicillin right away. It would do no harm if we were wrong but would stop the syphilis bacteria – the delicate, corkscrew-shaped *treponema pallida* – from nibbling away even more of his brain if we were right. 'Oh, you psychiatrists are always coming up with these far-fetched smart-Alec diagnoses', said the physician. 'Look. He's Irish and he's got some tremor. They say he only has a pint or two a day but I bet it's a lot more than that. He's probably got *delirium tremens*.' (DTs – literally 'the shaking delirium' that occurs in a minority of heavy and daily drinkers after they suddenly stop drinking or sharply reduce their alcohol intake.)

The next day, laboratory results started arriving. The routine blood tests were pretty normal but the CSF contained quite a few white cells, which shouldn't happen with simple DTs and within a few hours, there were excited phone calls from the bacteriology department, for whom this was a bit of a treat since nearly all cases of syphilis were diagnosed and treated at specialized Sexually Transmitted Disease clinics, which our hospital didn't have. All tests for syphilis were strongly positive in both blood and CSF. I ordered lots of penicillin. Typically, GPI has an insidious onset and by the time the diagnosis is made, a lot of brain cells have been destroyed. With penicillin or other antibiotics, the progression of the disease can always be halted but patients are still sometimes too badly damaged to be able to return to work. The unusually rapid onset in this case meant that we might nip it in the bud and that brain cells that were damaged but not dead would start working again. Without penicillin, Fergus would have progressed in a few months to the sort of uncommunicative apathy that typifies the last stages of all dementias. Within a few days, he was emerging from his delirium and able to fill a few important gaps in the history.

Before the war, he had been in the regular army and his postings in the service of King and Empire included a period in the Far East during the late 1930s. Like many a sex-starved squaddie, he patronised the local bordellos and got a dose of syphilis which was treated, in those pre-penicillin days, with Salvarsan, the first of medicine's 'magic bullets', discovered twenty years earlier. Unlike many pre-war remedies, Salvarsan probably wasn't entirely useless but if it worked at all, it often stunned rather than eliminated the *treponema*. Undamaged by the war itself, he easily made the transition to civilian life and marriage but here his robust health proved a disadvantage.

One reason that GPI is now so rarely seen in developed countries is that it is rare for people to get through life without having at least a few courses of penicillin or other antibiotics. So sensitive is *treponema pallida* to the right antibiotics that even a short course has a good chance of killing any lurking organisms, or at least sending them back to sleep for many more years. Most fortunately for mankind – and quite unlike the *gonococcus* that causes gonorrhoea – *treponema pallida* seems unable to develop the resistance to antibiotics that several other dangerous bacteria have mastered. Since this model employee had never felt ill enough to see his GP, he had therefore never taken penicillin. Now the bacteria had woken up good and proper and were clearly starting to behave like something out of a microscopic version of 'Alien'. After we cut short their little bit of fun, he made a good recovery and was back at work in less than three months, though he did have some permanent damage to the nerves of his legs.

There was just one delicate little diplomatic problem to be dealt with. Although syphilis affecting the brain isn't usually contagious, because there are no open sores or rashes, there was the worrying possibility that he had unknowingly infected his wife and, through her, his children. Fortunately, the family were either trusting and uncurious or, if they suspected the real nature of his illness, they didn't want to talk about it – probably the former. We certainly didn't tell them (in those days, we were allowed to exercise our discretion) and it wasn't difficult to disguise the truth by talking vaguely about his having had a 'tropical illness'. They were happy to give us blood samples. All were negative.

APPENDIX 2
Flow-chart for decision-making.

Before you reach 50, think about death and dementia, since one is certain and the other not unlikely. Make a living will/advance decision that specifically includes your dementia preferences and make sure your GP and family know about it.

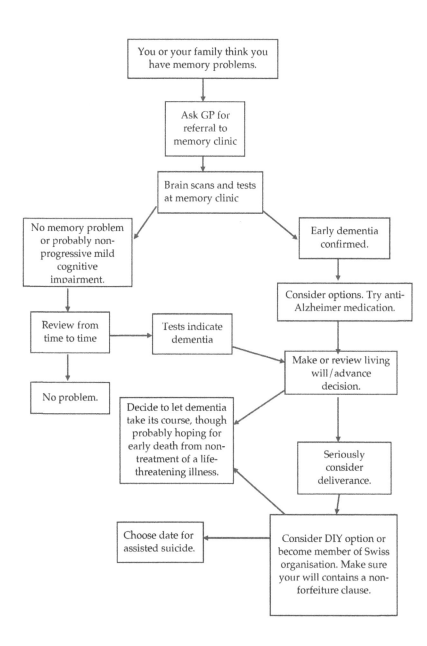

APPENDIX 3
Useful Addresses and Contacts

For templates and advice about living wills/advance decisions:

Assisted Dying Assistance. (adassistance.org.uk)
and 01768 775566

Compassion in Dying. (compassionindying.org.uk/)

Free information line: 0800 999 2434

Other organisations:

Alzheimer Society UK. (www.alzheimers.org.uk/)

National dementia helpline 0300 222 11 22
Probably the best first port of call in the UK for information about dementias in general and facilities for dealing with them.

Lewy body dementia is related to Parkinson's disease and Parkinson's UK (www.parkinsons.org.uk/lewy-body) provides information about it.

The Huntington's disease association (www.hda.org.uk)

There is an organization specializing in progressive supranuclear palsy (PNP) and cortico-basal degeneration (CBD). (pspassociation.org.uk)

VASCULAR DEMENTIA.

The Stroke Association (www.stroke.org.uk) has good online information about vascular dementia.

MEDICALERT (www.medicalert.org.uk/)

For £32 a year (as of 2019) Medicalert will keep details of your important medical information, including a living will. Bracelets and dog-tags in a variety of materials and even specially-marked waterproof watches alert medical staff to your needs and wishes.

NICE

The National Institute For Health Care and Excellence

NICE provides guidelines about current 'best practice' aimed mainly at health-professionals but much of it should be reasonably understandable to the more general reader. In particular, guidelines for choosing the right first-line and second-line medications for the various types of dementia, as well as broader aspects of dementia care and management, can be found at:

nice.org.uk/search?q=alzheimer's%20disease

The information may also help you to understand why many doctors – even specialists – are increasingly reluctant to deviate from what are supposed to be guidelines but are often seen as rules.

British Right-to-Die societies

My Death, My Decision (mydeath-mydecision.org.uk/) its Scottish counterpart Friends at the End – FATE (friends-at-the-end.org.uk/) and End of Life Choices Jersey (facebook. com/endoflifechoicesjersey/) are the only British organisations campaigning for MAID legislation that is not restricted to patients expected to die anyway within six months. They are members of the Assisted Dying Coalition (secretariat@assisteddying.org.uk) which is supported by Humanists UK and Humanist Society Scotland.

Dignity in Dying (dignityindying.org.uk) currently restricts its campaigning to the legalization of MAID only for the terminally ill with a maximum life expectancy of six months.

Right-to-die societies in other countries.

The World Federation of Right-to-Die societies (worldrtd.net) has links to 53 organisations in 27 countries. It holds a bi-annual conference and gives details of other meetings, as well as news of progress and setbacks throughout the world.

The Samaritans. (www.samaritans.org)

It is customary to give a link to The Samaritans in any book or article that deals with suicide. I won't break with custom but I will make the point that the first and only major controlled study that claimed Samaritans reduced the suicide rate (towns with a Samaritan switchboard vs towns without one in the mid 1960s when telephoning outside one's own town was expensive) was soon refuted. That was because during the study period in the early 1960s, toxic coal-gas was gradually replaced, town by town, with non-toxic natural gas from the North Sea. Samaritan centres began to appear in the 1950s. The suicide rate fell sharply after 1963 but only because coal-gas suicides, which had long been the main method in Britain, gradually disappeared. Suicides using other methods either increased or stayed fairly steady, regardless of local Samaritan access.

APPENDIX 4

Specimen advance decision/ living will for dementia

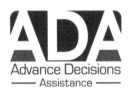

DEMENTIA VERSION
(Suitable for someone with a dementia diagnosis, or worried about dementia, and with other health problems.)

An ADA staff member has collaborated with the BMA in a YouTube lecture

(www.youtube.com/watch?v=yw66KHs1g_0&feature=youtu.be)

about the role of family and friends in decisions about various forms of tube-feeding in dementia and severe brain injury.

DAWN

Dawn is 82 years old and has just been diagnosed with Alzheimer's disease. She knows that this condition is progressive and wants to plan for the future. She does not want to live for years with dementia, or to die in its late stages. She enjoys her independence and is filled with horror at the thought of moving to a care home. Her adult daughter says she will be only too happy to care for her, but Dawn doesn't want to be a burden to her daughter.

Dawn also has high blood pressure, angina and heart problems and is at risk of having a heart attack or stroke. She hopes that by refusing treatment for her heart problems – as well as refusing to be resuscitated - she may die sooner of a heart attack or stroke than she would of dementia. She has discussed her Advance Decision with her daughter, who is very distressed that her mother is unwilling to live as long as is medically possible.

Dawn's Advance Decision:

When I am unable to make or communicate decisions about my medical treatment, I wish to refuse all treatments/interventions which may prolong my life. This refusal includes (but is not limited to):

- Cardio-pulmonary resuscitation (CPR)

- Ventilation

- Treatments designed to maintain or replace a vital bodily function
  (such as a heart pacemaker)

- A feeding tube

- Antibiotics given for a potentially life-threatening infection

- Specialised treatments for particular conditions
  (such as chemotherapy, dialysis, or insulin)

- Current treatments/medications
  statins, blood pressure medication, angina medication

I maintain this refusal even if my life is shortened as a result.

If I refuse food and/or drink by mouth, I refuse repeated attempts to feed/hydrate me; or being persuaded or cajoled to eat and/or drink – even if this refusal shortens my life.

I do consent to treatment to alleviate pain or distress, even if it shortens my life.

I should like to die at home in my own bed, even if this shortens my life. I do not want to be rushed to hospital in my final days or hours.

Important note:

Because I have recently been diagnosed with dementia (Alzheimer's Disease), I have attached a statement from my GP confirming that at the time of completing this Advance Decision, I have the mental capacity to make the decisions contained in it.

Signature & date

Witness signature & date

'Advance Values Statement':

I am writing this Advance Decision in order to plan for the future, as best I can in an uncertain world. I have recently been diagnosed with dementia (Alzheimer's Disease), and know that this will be progressive. However, I hope to avoid years of declining mental capacity, followed by a lingering death from advanced-stage dementia. I should prefer to die sooner, while I can still engage fully in, and take pleasure from, the aspects of life that I value. And I should like to die at home, in my own bed, if possible. I do not want to be rushed into hospital in my final days or hours.

The things that are important to me are my independence (I still live in my own home, with some occasional help), my social life (I am a member of several clubs and societies and have a small circle of good friends), and my hobbies (regular visits to the theatre and cinema, and volunteering for the National Trust). I am filled with horror at the prospect of moving into a care home and the restrictions and institutionalisation that would involve. Although my daughter has offered to care for me, I do not want to move in with my daughter and son-in-law when I can no longer look after myself. I don't want to be a burden to her, particularly as she has a demanding job involving a lot of travel. I am well aware how much of a burden caring for an elderly relative with dementia can be: my niece did it for her aunt (my sister) in similar circumstances, and it nearly split the family apart.

I have a number of other health problems – high blood pressure, angina, and heart weakness and arrhythmia – and I am at high risk of having a stroke or heart attack. I have written my Advance Decision to refuse all treatments for these conditions, including resuscitation, once I am no longer able to make medical decisions for myself. My hope is that I may die sooner of a heart attack or stroke than I will of dementia, and that this will happen while I am still enjoying at least some of the things that are important to me, and before I need full-time care in an institution. For this reason, I have refused the medications I am currently taking for my heart and other problems, once I cannot make or communicate my own decisions about medication. I also do not want to be given any further specialised medications for these conditions (or any other medical conditions I might develop after losing my decision-making capacity). And, just in case I do not die of a heart attack or stroke, I have also refused the treatments and interventions that are common in late-stage dementia: antibiotics and a feeding tube. Please also note that I do not want to be 'force fed', however kindly.

Finally, I should perhaps mention that my daughter is very distressed that I am thinking about my death, and about the contents of this Advance Decision, which I have discussed with her – it seems she wants me to live for ever! I understand her feelings but please don't let her wishes overrule what I've written here. This is my life and my choice. I am sorry to cause her pain and distress and hope that in time she will be able to overcome this, with the help of my son-in-law, who fully respects my choices. I know what I want to happen and I am settled in these wishes.

Attached statement from a health practitioner (e.g. GP, dementia nurse, psychiatric social worker, IMCA)

I have discussed the content of this Advance Decision with ... Dawn X ... and I am satisfied that she has the mental capacity to make the decisions contained in it. She understands what she is signing, has weighed the pros and cons of these decisions, and can remember that s/he has made them.

Name: Dr................................

Signature: .... Date: ......

Role & contact information: e.g. GP, surgery address

....

APPENDIX 5

Blank Advance Decision/ Living Will

T he next section is a real Advance Decision/Living Will form, reproduced by kind permission of Advance Decisions Assistance. If you haven't already made an Advance Decision, you may photocopy the next three pages and fill in the relevant details. It will be helpful if you add your own 'value statement' at the end on the third sheet, by hand or using a printer and pasting the text. You should then make and sign several copies that can be given to family members, close friends, your GP, your lawyer, Health Care Attorney and anyone else who may need to know your wishes. It is advisable to confirm the instructions - and if appropriate, revise them - from time to time and re-circulate them with an additional signature and date, especially if many years have passed since you first completed the form. That will discourage interventionist medical and nursing staff from arguing that you may have changed your mind in the intervening period.

```
┌─────────────┐
│ AFFIX A     │
│ PASSPORT    │
│ PHOTO       │
│ HERE        │
└─────────────┘
```

ADVANCE DECISION FORM (VERSION D)

This version is most suitable for someone with a recent diagnosis of dementia, or worried about dementia, and with other health problems.

Note to person completing this form: If this version is not quite right for you, remember that you can personalise it by adding or deleting information. You may also like to look at the other versions on the ADA website: www.adassistance.org.uk Further information can also be found on the website; or phone us if you have any questions: 01757 289453

This Advance Decision is intended to apply indefinitely unless I specifically revoke it. I give permission for anyone legitimately involved in my care to read it.

Your name (block capitals):

_____

Your address:

_____

_____

Your date of birth: _____

Your NHS no. (if known): _____

Your GP's name & address:

_____

_____

Statement for you to sign:

When I am unable to make or communicate decisions about my medical treatment, I wish to REFUSE all treatments/interventions which may prolong my life.

This refusal includes (but is not limited to):

- Cardio-pulmonary resuscitation (CPR)

- Ventilation

- Treatments designed to maintain or replace a vital bodily function
(such as a heart pacemaker)

- A feeding tube

- Antibiotics given for a potentially life-threatening infection

- Specialised treatments for particular conditions
(such as chemotherapy, dialysis, or insulin)

- Other current treatments/medications (if relevant) - say what these are:

_____

_____

_____

I maintain this refusal even if it shortens my life.

If I refuse food and/or drink by mouth, I refuse repeated attempts to feed/hydrate me;

or being persuaded or cajoled to eat or drink – even if this refusal shortens my life.

I do consent to treatment to alleviate pain or distress, even if it shortens my life.

Your signature: _____ Date: _____

Witness signature: _____ Date: _____

Witness name & address:

_____

_____

_____

(Delete note below if you have NOT been diagnosed with dementia.)

Important note:

Because I have recently been diagnosed with dementia, I have attached a statement from a health practitioner confirming that at the time of completing this Advance Decision, I have the mental capacity to make the decisions contained in it.

[This 'mental capacity statement' – is also available on the ADA website, or we can send it to you if you phone us on the number above.]

Advance Values Statement:

You may choose (but do not need to) to include a further short statement here. This can explain the decisions you have made and what is important to you. You can add pages as necessary.

[There are some examples of Advance Values Statements on the ADA website.]

Acknowledgements

Board members at My Death, My Decision, (MDMD), read earlier drafts and made several suggestions but the views expressed in the book are my own and not those of MDMD. However, our views are close in many respects. MDMD campaigns (as I do) for Medical Assistance in Dying to be available to 'all mentally competent adults with incurable health problems that reduce their quality of life permanently below the level they are willing to accept, provided this is their own, well considered, persistent request', including those with early stage dementia, before they lose the mental capacity to make a life-ending decision. I am, though, particularly grateful to Robert Ince – lately Convener of the Unitarian Church in Britain – for guiding me through the complex development of early Christianity's attitudes to suicide. Asunción Alvarez explained how Colombian MAID law developed. Prof. Norman Cantor allowed me to quote from one of his papers and from the latest version of his own living will. Iain Chalmers read and commented on the first draft with his characteristic thoroughness. Among my fellow-psychiatrists still in harness, Julian Bird and Justin Basquille helped to keep me up to date with current diagnostic and therapeutic trends. Julian also provides occasional second opinions for particularly complex patients wanting to go to Switzerland. Dr Martin Haraldsen explained Norway's system of nursing-home care and funding. Bert Keizer and Jenne Wielenga of the Levenseindekliniek explained recent Dutch developments. Sheila Kitzinger of Advance Decisions Assistance gave me permission to reproduce her organisation's forms and information about Advance Decisions. Alex Pandolfo has provided regular bulletins from his planned journey to Switzerland, where Silvan Luley and René Casanova at Dignitas and Dr Erika Preisig and Ruedi Habegger at LifeCircle are helpful front-line correspondents. I shared ideas over many conversations with Daniel Simpson and with Emmanuel Streel, my co-author in several addiction publications. At Louvain University, he was a student of Gabriel Ringlet, whose book he translated for me. The historian and novelist Gillian Tindall and my publisher Karl Sabbagh tried – not always successfully - to discourage some of my more strongly-expressed feelings about obstructions to choice and compassion in dying based on religious dogmas.

The dozen or so dementia patients for whom I did Capacity and psychiatric assessments for their assisted deaths in Switzerland taught me a lot, not just about the effects of dementia on them and their families but also about the levels of altruism, love and friendship that human beings can achieve and inspire and their ability to face the conundrum of death with courage, coolness and humour.

I attended two international 'end of life' conferences while writing this book. At the last one, held in Ghent early in March this year, I met academics and clinicians from every inhabited continent who presented the very latest in end-of-life research. Canadians were particularly prominent and I thank Stefanie Green, the president of CAMAP – the Canadian Association of MAID Assessors and Providers – for sharing her experiences. Aida Dehkhoda from New Zealand and Joachim Cohen of

Belgium kindly let me have their slides. Ginette Bravo of Quebec kept me posted about research and developments in that Province.

A special mention must be made of Dr Michael Irwin, former medical director of the United Nations, whom I have known since we were both committee members of the Voluntary Euthanasia Society, which he later chaired. (We are also alumni of the same ancient medical school – St Bartholomew's Hospital.) He went on to found SOARS - the Society for Old-Age Rational Suicide, which became My Death, My Decision in 2015. He has donated generously to the cause and also funded the National Secular Society's 'Secularist of the Year' award from 2005 to 2017. Among many other notable achievements, he once - without revealing its nature - gave Margaret Thatcher placebo medication when she demanded antibiotics for a very ordinary cold that did not need them during a visit to the UN building in 1984. She was apparently very grateful for his personal and attentive treatment. Some of the passages in this book are taken or adapted from the 2015 essay collection *I'll See Myself Out, Thank You*, which we co-edited. At 88, he shows no signs of wanting to leave the stage but hopes to do so with dignity and his usual panache when the time is right.

Most of my nearly two hundred footnotes refer to publications by a legion of 'pure' academics and academically-inclined clinicians in medicine, nursing and psychology who often devote some of their unpaid leisure time to the critical and sceptical pursuit of truth in a tradition that goes back at least to Aristotle. We should all be grateful for their contributions to knowledge, as we should for the public-spirited founders and helpers of Wikipedia, which provided a small number of sole references but also several useful links to more detailed academic sources of information.

Normally, people who provide information, criticisms, insights or suggestions for a book are delighted to be mentioned in the acknowledgements section. It tells us something about the atmosphere surrounding the Medical Assistance in Dying debate that four doctors whose help was particularly welcome requested anonymity. One is an old-age psychiatrist – encountered quite by chance during a music weekend - who provided extensive and valuable comment. Two are from palliative care.

Colin Brewer.
London, April 2019.

About the Author

B orn in Sunderland, Dr Colin Brewer qualified in 1963. After working as a ship's surgeon and a GP, he specialised in psychiatry. As a lecturer and research fellow at Birmingham University, he published studies on obesity, social work, abortion and puerperal psychosis and was psychiatric advisor to the British Pregnancy Advisory Service and the University Health Service. Noticing that he had also published a much-cited paper on alcoholic brain damage, colleagues happily referred their alcoholic patients, so he became an alcoholism specialist as well. Later, as director of the alcoholism service at Westminster Hospital, he pioneered rapid, economical withdrawal for heroin addicts under sedation, and treatment with the heroin-blocking drug naltrexone. This became so popular that he left the NHS in 1987 and set up the Stapleford Centre, Britain's only private or NHS clinic that offered opiate addicts a choice between humane withdrawal or methadone maintenance. Since the British addiction Establishment strongly opposed methadone for two decades despite growing evidence, this caused conflicts that were a factor in his appearance, with six other Stapleford doctors, before the General Medical Council in 2005.

He was erased from the medical register but the clinic continues under a former colleague, offering similar services. The *Daily Telegraph's* Mick Brown wrote a very critical account of the Establishment's persecution that can be viewed, with Dr Brewer's own perspective, at his website <u>planetservetus. org</u>. From the 1970s, he wrote articles (some about medically-assisted dying) for the *Guardian, Times, Independent, New Society, New Scientist, Spectator* and *World Medicine*, as well as a regular column in *General Practitioner*. In 2007, he conceived and co-produced a play *(The Last Priest)* at the Edinburgh Festival and Islington's King's Head Theatre about post-Classical Europe's first self-identified atheist, the 17th-century village priest Jean Meslier.

He is a board member of My Death, My Decision and the convener of its medical group.

Index

A

Abled, vs disabled 144
Abortion, changes in attitude of GMC to 231
Abortion, differences between north and south Italy 127
Abortion, illegal in S America 142
Abortion, numbers in Britain 141
Abortions, back-street, rapid disappearance of after legalisation 210
Active euthanasia 74, 103
Advance care planning 98
Advance decision 44, 45, 74
Advance Directive 44, 183
Advance directive, and withdrawing nutrition 158
Advance Euthanasia Directive 186
Advanced dementia 37, 150
Advanced dementia, and insomnia 102
Afro-American attitudes to assisted dying 125
Ageism 73
Agitation 40
Agitation, failure to reduce 108
Ahmedzai, Prof Sam, and support for MAID 151-2, 155
Aikenhead, Thomas, execution for atheism 120
Alcohol consumption, and dementia 32

Alcohol consumption, and inability to dress 54
Alcoholics Anonymous 128
"All good doctors do it anyway" 86
Alton, Lord, and anti-abortion activism 131
Alton, Lord, awarded Sacred Military Constantinian Order of St George 131
Alvarez, Al, book The Savage God 116
Alving, Osvald, fictional character 15, 33, 173
Alzheimer Society UK 16
Alzheimer, Professor Alois 38
Alzheimer's Disease International 151
Alzheimer's Society 106
Alzheimer's, and bad driving 50
Alzheimer's, and disorientation 54
Alzheimer's, and inappropriate sexual behaviour 62
Alzheimer's, and increased alcohol consumption 58
Alzheimer's, and lack of insight 57
Alzheimer's, and neuropsychiatric symptoms 40
Alzheimer's, average duration 16
Alzheimer's, drugs for 27
Alzheimer's, increased effects of alcohol 55

Alzheimer's, increased risk with age 49
Alzheimer's, rate of progression 30
Ambivalence, about MAID in families
    157
Ambivalence, in medical and nursing
    staff 158, 159
American Association of Suicidology,
    (position statement) 21
Amitriptyline, in pain relief 221
Amputees, inability of God to heal 172
Andrews, June, Professor 121
Anencephaly 190
Angels 23
Anschluss, high Jewish suicide rate
    following 177
Antenatal diagnosis 191
Antenatal diagnosis, and incidence of
    congenital abnormalities 191
Antenatal testing 193
Antibiotic treatment, inappropriate 102
Antibiotic treatment, for pneumonia 98
Antibiotics, intravenous 161
Antidepressants 40, 52, 155
Antidepressants, as inappropriate
    response 205
Anxiety 39
Apathy 40
APOE, testing for 168
Apolipoprotein-E (APOE). 166
Arteriosclerotic dementia 31
Aspirin, unsuitability for suicide 212
Assisted dying, ethnic differences in
    attitude to 92
Association of Palliative Medicine 156
Atheroma 30
Atlee, Clement 50
Atrophy, of brain in Alzheimer demen-
    tia 28, 30
Attempted murder, failure to prosecute
    author 90
Augustine, Saint 117
Auschwitz 133
Australia, Federal parliament overturns
    NT law 22
Autonomy 212
Autonomy, of patients 136, 137
Axons 28

B

Babies for Burning, film 143fn
Badham, Paul, Rev Professor 116
Baird, Sir Dugald, and abortion 232
BAME respondents to survey 122
Barrington, Mary-Rose, coins 'self-de-
    liverance' 214
Basal ganglia 33
Beatles, The 72
Beckett, Samuel 177
Bedsores 99, 159
Belgium 24, 129
Belgium, Muslim attitudes to MAID
    in 124
Belgium, palliative care physicians
    active in law reform 153
Belgium, possible acceptance of UK
    patients in 206
Belsen, concentration camp 17
Benelux countries 25
Benevolent paternalism 91
Bennett, Alan 42
Bennett, Alan, and blue urine 42
Berlin, Sir Isaiah 138
"Best interest", of patients 84
Bible, neutral about suicide 116
Bipolar illness 35, 40, 41
Birth control 195
Blair, Tony 16
Bland, Tony, 83
Bland, Tony, and persistent vegetative
    state 80
BMJ (see British Medical Journal)
Braga, Council of 117
Brain cells 28
Brain scans 222
Brain tumours 35
Brain, and information processing 38
Brain, diagram of 29
Brassington, Ian 134, 144
British Medical Journal (BMJ), survey
    hacked by opponents 130
Browne-Wilkinson, Lord, judge 80, 81
Buchman, Dr Sandy, president-elect of
    Canadian Medical Association 153,
    154
Buchman, Dr Sandy, changes opinion
    on MAID 153

Buddhism 119
Bureaucrats, monstrous regiment of 241

C

Caesarean section, increased use of 194
Calvin, John, and execution of Miguel
   Servetus 120
Campaigns for change in the law 70
Camus, Albert 179
Canada 24, 154
Canada, palliative care physicians sup-
   port for MAID 153
Canada, Medical Assistance in Dying
   (MAID), 182
Cancer patients, with psychiatric
   history 221
Cantor, Norman 109, 110
Cardiac arrest 23
Cardio-pulmonary resuscitation (CPR),
   inappropriate use of 242
Cardio-pulmonary resuscitation (CPR),
   poor outcomes in elderly 242
Carey, Lord, former archbishop, and
   support for MAID 117
Carmelite nun, requests euthanasia 129
Catechism, Roman Catholic Church
   115
Catholic Bishops Conference of Eng-
   land and Wales 132
Catholic Church of New Zealand 132
Catholic Trust for England and Wales
   132
Cavities, in brain. (See also Ventricles)
   30
Cerebral cortex 28
Cerebral hemispheres, functions of 28
Cerebro-spinal fluid 29
Champagne suicide case 84
Childbirth 190
Christianity, opposition to assisted
   dying 115
Chromosomes 166
Church of England Synod, changes
   canon law 116
Church of England, attitudes to
   suicide 5
Circumcision, infant, no recollection
   of 143

Codicils 45
Coercion, fear of 161
Coercion, to remain alive 161-2
Cognition 41
Cohen, Nick 133
Coil (intrauterine contraceptive device)
   142
Colombia 132, 153
Colombia, attitudes to assisted dying 22
"Comfort measures only" orders 100
Confucianism 119
Conscientiousness, protective effect
   of 170
Conservative, MPs voting on assisted
   dying 119
Constipation 99
Contented Dementia Trust 106
Coroner, not necessary to involve after
   MAID in Switzerland 223
Cortico-basal degeneration 32
Costs, of dementia care 199
Costs, of nursing homes in UK 202
Counselling, for family members 8
Cranial decompression surgery 97
Cremation 138
Cremation, included in cost of MAID
   in Switzerland 222
Cremation, vs returning body to UK
   from Switzerland 223
Creutzfeld-Jakob disease 33
Crossroad burial, of suicides 116
CT scan 30
Curare, use in MAID after uncon-
   sciousness 155

D

Dalrymple, Dr Theodore 239
Daniels, Dr Anthony 239
Data Protection Act 1998 229
Dawson, Lord 86
Dawson, Lord, and clinical discretion
   241
Dawson, Lord, and euthanasia of King
   George V 86-87
Deafness, congenital 144
Death, fear of 1
Death, medicated, advantages of 238

Death, need to accept inevitability of 205

De Duve, Prof. Christian 128

Degenerative diseases, co-existing with dementia 150

Dehydration 81, 219, 220

Dehydration, death from 18, 158

Dehydration, nobody survives unrelieved 79

Deliverance 24, 105, 148

Deliverance tourism 206

Deliverance, after losing Capacity 145

Deliverance, before losing Capacity 145

Deliverance, meaning of 21

Dementia directive 110

Dementia pugilistica 32

Dementia, aggression in 27

Dementia, and falls 51

Dementia, and hypersexuality 44

Dementia, and identity 44

Dementia, and infidelity 44

Dementia, and paedophilia 44

Dementia, and personhood 44

Dementia, and police attention 44

Dementia, and promiscuity 44

Dementia, as madness 41

Dementia, as mental or psychiatric illness 13, 41

Dementia, commonest cause of death in England and Wales 13

Dementia, degenerative type 28

Dementia, delusions in 27

Dementia, early 145

Dementia, hallucinations in 27

Dementia, mood changes in 27

Dementia, psychotic symptoms in 27

Dementia, reversible causes of 35

Denial 66, 157

Denning, Lord Justice 115

Denning, Lord Justice, absurdity of criminalising assisting suicide 238

Department of Health, advice on sedation in spina bifida 244

Depression 39

Depression, as understandable reaction to diagnosis 52

Depression, presumed disturbance in brain chemistry 39

Depression, understandable 39

Depression, as inappropriate diagnosis 205

Depressive illness 35, 40, 41

Deter, Frau Auguste 38

Dialysis 73

Diamorphine 52

Dignitas 4, 6, 12, 52, 53

Dignitas, and early dementia 206

Dignity in Dying (DiD) 93, 152, 189, 236

Dignity in Dying, survey on funding of opposition to MAID 129

Dimbleby Lecture, BBC 39

Director of Public Prosecutions (DPP) 90, 137, 216, 223

Director of Public Prosecutions (DPP), recent advice to doctors 229-30

Disability lobby 142, 143, 145, 192

Disability lobby, attitude to antenatal testing and abortion 194

Disability, medical or 'tragedy' model 189

Disability, social model of 189

Disability, and terminology 189

Discrimination, protection against 144

Distress, levels of when nutrition withdrawn 159

"Do not hospitalise" orders 99

"Do not resuscitate" orders (DNR) 73, 100, 160

"Do-It-Yourself" suicide 22

Dobbin, Jim, MP 119

Doctor-administered medication, preference for 24

Doctors, privileges of 7, 14

Doctors, self-deliverance among 235

Doctors, trust in 241

Documents, and visual or neurological impairments in writing or signing 207

Donne, John 177, 214

Double Effect, doctrine of 79

Down syndrome 144, 190

Down syndrome, and termination of affected pregnancies 191

Down syndrome, large reduction in incidence 191

Down syndrome, desirability of children with 144
Down syndrome, difference vs abnormality 189
Down syndrome, taboo about discussing negative aspects 193
Down syndrome, and persisting need for clinical services 192
Drugs, stupefying, alternatives to in self-deliverance 212
Dutch doctors, held in high esteem 185
Dutch doctors, most trusted and highly regarded 146

E

Early dementia, normal life and 36
Early dementia, preservation of mental capacity in 36
Eastern Orthodox Christianity, and suicide 119
Economy, burden on 201
Embryo selection 195
End of Life (EOL), decisions 157-8
Epictetus 214
Epidural anaesthesia 194
Epilepsy 40
Episiotomy 194
Ethics committees 243
Ethnicity, and differences in Alzheimer risk 170
European Commission on Human Rights 226
Evangelical Protestantism in USA 118
'Everything must be done', responses to those who request that 208
Excommunication, of suicides 70
Exit 211
Extended family, changes in 88

F

Facebook, use for surveys 95
Facial cancer, failure of palliative care in 129
Fear of developing dementia 64, 95
Fear, of becoming burden 109
Fertilisation 142

Final solution, and Nazis 174
Financial considerations, in dementia care 76
Finlay, Baroness 132
Folic acid, and neural tube defects 191
Fore tribe, New Guinea, and prion disease 33
Free Presbyterian Church of Scotland 131
Froggatt, Dr Gordon 154-5
Frontal lobes, importance of 28
Fronto-temporal dementia 28, 32

G

Gawande, Atul 88, 196
Gene modification in Huntington's disease 33
General Medical Council (GMC) 208
General Medical Council, published guidance 226-9
General Paresis of the Insane (GPI) 14, 15, 16, 36
General Practitioner magazine 91
Genes, dominant 166
Genes, in Huntington's disease 167
Genes, recessive 167
Genetic testing 27, 195
Genetics, of Alzheimer's 166
George III, King, and Alzheimer's 43
George III, King, did not have porphyria 42
George V, King, dies by euthanasia 86-7
German law, legality of assisted suicide since 1920s 24
Goebbels, Joseph and Magda, kill themselves and their children 176
Grant, Brenda, and failure to observe living will 81
Greek Orthodox 127
Greek Orthodox Church, and cremation 139
Gulf States, and futile treatment 124

H

Haemorrhage, brain 30
Hallucinations 39, 67

Hallucinations, frightening, in dementia 200

Happiness, in dementia 200

Harvey, William, suicide kit 13

Head trauma, as cause of Alzheimer's 32

Health Care Power of Attorney 160, 161

Health Professionals for Assisted Dying (HPAD) 152

Heath, Edward 50

Heroin addicts 123

Heterozygous 167

Hillsborough football disaster 80

Hinduism 119

Hippocampus 29

HIV, and prejudice against homosexuality 82

Holocaust 176

Homozygous 167

Hospices 147

House of Lord, bishops in 117

Huntington's chorea 33

Huntington's Disease 17, 28, 32, 33, 49, 158, 166, 189

Huntington's Disease, 50% of offspring at risk 33

Huntington's Disease, abortion in 34

Huntington's Disease, and embryo selection 34, 192

Huntington's Disease, and withdrawing nutrition 79

Huntington's Disease, increased risk of suicide 34

Huntington's Disease, low uptake of genetic testing for 34, 167, 178

Huntington's Disease, misdiagnosed as hysteria 39

Hydration, artificial 72

Hypothyroidism 35

I

I'll See Myself Out, Thank You (book) 21fn, 152

Ibsen, Henrik 15

Iceland, and Down syndrome 145

Immigration, attitudes to 144

Implantation, of embryo 142

Incompetent patients, and continuous deep sedation 183

Incompetent patients, and MAID 183

Infarction 30

Inquest, avoidance of, after MAID in Switzerland 223

Inquisition, Holy, and homicide 120

Insight, and frontal lobe atrophy 57

Insight, loss of 40

Intensive care units (ICU) 123

Intensive care units (ICU), influence of religion on treatment 127

International Association for Hospice and Palliative Care 149

Intrauterine Contraceptive Device (IUD) 142

Intrauterine Contraceptive Device, as abortifacient 142

Intravenous medication, preference for in MAID 24

Intravenous medication, preferred by 99.9% in Canada 155

Involuntary euthanasia 79

IQ, protective effect of high 169

Irwin, Dr Michael 21, 231

Islam, and cremation 139

Islam, and organ donation 125

Islam, attitudes to assisted dying 124

Islam, attitudes to suicide 118

Islam, beliefs about afterlife 125

J

Jackson, Michael 155

Johnson, Harriet McBryde 193

Johnson, Samuel, Dr 129

Johnson, Samuel, Dr, and fear of death 178

Junior doctors, lacking confidence in crises 87

Justinian, Code of 119

K

Koestler, Arthur 190, 213

Korsakov syndrome 32

L

Labour Party, voting on assisted dying 119
Last sacrament 114
Latino, attitudes to assisted dying 125
Lewy body dementia 32, 37, 48, 154
Liberal Democrats, voting on assisted dying 119
LifeCircle 4, 6, 217
LifeCircle, and early dementia 206
LifeCircle, intravenous infusion 23
Living and Dying Well, secretive about religious links 130-132
Living will 44, 45, 73, 74, 93, 109,
Living wills, and avoidance of assisted feeding 208
Living wills, importance of unambiguous instructions in 187
Lobotomy, beneficial effects of 44
Loneliness, in old age 196
Longevity, and increased incidence of degenerative diseases 196
Lung disease, and difficulty of palliation 211
Lyall, Bernard, and Katherine Whitehorn 163-4
Lying, by carers and family 46
Lyme disease 35

M

M.P.s, influence of religion on voting 119
Machismo 141
Mackay, Lord 131
Mad cow disease 33
Madness and dementia 41
MAID (see Medical Assistance in Dying)
Mania 39
Manic depressive illness 14
Margolyes, Miriam 215
Marsh, Henry 12, 16, 89, 122, 234
Marsh, Henry, and persistent vegetative state 96
Marsh, Henry, suicide kit 11
Maternal mortality 195
Maugham, Somerset 115

Maximalism, therapeutic 209
May, Theresa, and dementia tax 200
Mechanical ventilation 73
Médecins Sans Frontières 105
Medical Assistance in Dying (MAID) 21, 151
Medical Assistance in Dying (MAID), and spiritual comfort 128
Medical Assistance in Dying (MAID), may be seen as cowardice 173
Medical Defence Union, and advice to doctors 229
Medical notes, and Scottish law 222
Medical notes, appeals against refusal of 222
Medical notes, obtaining 222
Medical notes, right to access 46
Medical Protection Society, and advice to doctors 229
Medical records, obtaining 214
Medical reports, needed for Swiss organisations 206
Medically-assisted suicide 11
Medically-Assisted Rational Suicide (MARS) 19, 22
Medico-philosophical collectives 242
Mediterranean diet, possible protective effect of 169
Memory clinic 53, 205
Memory impairment 38
Mental Capacity 4, 24, 25, 3, 45, 93, 136, 145, 204, 222
Mental Capacity Act 2005 12
Mental Capacity, assessments, 30-day period in applications for dementia 206
Mental Capacity, definitions 12
Midazolam, use of in MAID 52, 155
Mild cognitive impairment (MCI) 48, 53
Mini mental state examination (MMSE) 50, 52, 68
Mini-stroke 30
Miracles 172
Moderate dementia, and employment 36
Moderate dementia, and institutional care 36

Monotheism, and opposition to obstetric anaesthesia and birth control 195
Morphine 15, 82, 83, 140, 235, 236
Morphine, and doctrine of 'double effect' 79
Morphine, and informal use by GPs 234
Motor Neurone Disease 6
Motor Neurone Disease, and difficulty of travelling 204
Motor Neurone Disease, and signing documents 207
Motor Neurone Disease, fall in voluntary euthanasia for in Netherlands 178
MRI scan 30
Multiple sclerosis 41, 135, 144
Multiple systems atrophy 181
Munthe, Axel 114
Murray, Douglas 137, 138, 141, 143
Mustill, Lord, judge 80
My Death, My Decision 93, 180, 189, 236, 265

N

Nepal 122
Nerve fibres 30
Netherlands 22, 24
Netherlands, and case of Mrs A 186
Netherlands, palliative care physicians support for MAID 153
Netnography, in New Zealand 94
Neural tube defects (NTDs) 190
Neural tube defects (NTDs), changes in incidence 191
Neurodevelopment 143
Neurologist, personal account of Alzheimer's 68
Neuropsychiatric, conditions in dementia 41
Nicklinson, Tony 117, 180
Nietszche, Friedrich 180
Non-beneficial treatment 101
Non-prescription medication 24
Northern Territory (NT) Australia, first to legalise MAID 22
Norway, and palliative care challenges 148
Norway, and payment for dementia care 202

Not Dead Yet 193
Nursing homes, costs of in UK 202
Nutrition, artificial 72

O

Obsessional behaviour 39
Obstetric anaesthesia, changes in attitudes to 194
Obstetric practice, changes in 190
Oesophagus, tumour of 111
Old Commonwealth Anglosphere, attitudes to assisted dying 22
Omid T (patient) 181
Oral medication v. injected 23
Oregon 140
Oregon, palliative care physicians support for MAID 153
Orthodox Judaism, and cremation 139

P

Pain, in advanced dementia 99
Palliative care 6, 140, 148
Palliative care, barriers to in dementia 150
Palliative care, British, over-representation of religious doctors in 152
Palliative care, failing in pain relief 149
Palliative care, mission statement 149
Palliative care, risk to careers of MAID-supporting British consultants 156
Pandolfo, Alex, and early dementia 69
Pandolfo, Alex, and inappropriate diagnosis of depression 70
Pangloss, Dr 16
Paracetamol, unsuitability for suicide 212
Paraplegia 144
Parkinson's disease 33, 154
Parkinsonism 41
Parliament, atheists allowed to be members 140
Parliament, Catholics allowed to be members 140
Parliament, Jews allowed to be members 140
Parliament, U.K. 25

Parris, Matthew 89, 145, 165, 207, 209
Parris, Matthew, and dementia tax 200
Passive euthanasia 74, 103
Patient autonomy 91
Pensions, and dementia care 202
Pentecostal Christianity, in Afro-Caribbean communities 119
Pentobarbitone 24
Pentobarbitone, and patient survival after swallowing inadequate dose 217
Perception 41
Percutaneous Endoscopic Gastrostomy (PEG) 17, 72
Percutaneous Endoscopic Gastrostomy (PEG), and aspiration pneumonia 77
Percutaneous Endoscopic Gastrostomy (PEG), and physical restraint 77
Percutaneous Endoscopic Gastrostomy (PEG), Israeli study 75
Percutaneous Endoscopic Gastrostomy (PEG), Japanese study 75
Persistent vegetative state 18
Personality, changes in dementia 39, 43, 199
Personality, new versus old 44
Philosophers, existential, and suicide 179
Philosophy, differences in personal 171
Pick's disease 32
Placebo effect 28, 52
Pneumonia 159
Pneumonia, "the old man's friend" 97
Poets, high suicide rate of 179
Police, involvement of in dementia 215, 223
Post-mortem, brain changes in dementia 30
Pratchett, Terry 39
Pre-implantation diagnosis 145
Pre-natal screening, and discussion in disability context 192
Pre-natal testing 144
Pregnancy 190
Pre-senile dementia 49
Pressure ulcers 99
Pressure, from family members to 'do something' 160
Priestley, Rev. Joseph 65

Prion brain disease 33
Progressive supra-nuclear palsy 32
Propofol, use in MAID 155
Proxies, limited ability of to predict patient's wishes 161
Proxy, nomination of in Living Wills 160
Psychiatric evaluation, may be needed in Switzerland 221
Psychological tests, of brain function 222
Psychologists, clinical, and capacity assessment 222
Psychosis, inappropriate diagnosis of in dementia 225
Psychotherapy, and family members after MAID 8

Q

Quadriplegia 144
Quebec, citizens' views on voluntary euthanasia in dementia 181
Quebec, medication must be doctor-administered 182
Quebec, nurses' attitudes 145
Quebec, opinion surveys 15

R

Rational suicide in the elderly (book) 240
Refusal of treatment 74
Registrar of Births and Deaths 223
Religion, special importance in USA 22
Resources, desire not to waste 104
Respiration, distressing continuation after oral pentobarbitone 23
Ringlet, Gabriel 128
Risk Evaluation and Education for Alzheimer's Disease (REVEAL) 168
Risk, acceptance of impossibility to eliminate 146
Road deaths, changes in attitudes to 139
Robeck, Johan 115

S

Sabbagh, Karl 215
Samaritans 253
Saunders, Cicely, Dame, view of suicide 118
Saunders, Ernest, and unique recovery from Alzheimer's 172
Scales, Prunella 211
Schizophrenia 14, 41
Schizophrenia, low marriage rate in 41
Schumann, Robert 15
Scotland, and publication of first self-deliverance guide 213-4
Scott, Glen, and 'Glenn's last tape' 215
Sedation, generous, need for when nutrition withdrawn 158, 208
Self-deliverance 25, 144, 210, 212
Self-determination 182
Servetus, Miguel, Calvin executes for heresy 120
Severe dementia 37
Severe dementia, and feeding problems 37
Severe dementia, and incontinence 37
Severe dementia, and mental capacity 37
Severe dementia, and personal hygiene 37
Severely disabled, high standard of NHS and social services for 193
Sexual behaviour, inappropriate in dementia 43
Shakespeare and "Second Childhood" 104, 105
Shipman, Harold, and effects on medical practice 234
Shortness of breath, in advanced dementia 99
Shrinkage, of brain 28, 30
Singer, Peter 193
Sleep, lack of when nutrition withdrawn 159
Smythe, Dame Ethel 14
Social inhibitions, loss of 39
Social services, need for adequate 144
Society for Old-Age Rational Suicide (SOARS) 265

South Korea, attitudes to assisted dying 126
Spectator, The, describes cheerful seminar on self-deliverance 211
Spina bifida 144
Spina bifida, and advice from DHSS in 1978 about sedation 193
Spina bifida, and persisting disability 192
Spinsters, unlikely return of 200
Spiritual concerns, in advanced dementia 150
Spoon feeding 109
St Christopher's Hospice 150
State, and payment for dementia care 201
Stigma and mental illness 41
Stillbirths, and neural tube defects 191
Stroke 36
Subarachnoid haemorrhage 51
Sudden onset dementia 60
Suffering, alleged ennobling effects of 173
Suffering, anticipatory, immunity of dogs to 146
Suffering, existential 146
Suicide and mental illness 19
Suicide kit 11
Suicide, causes of "normal" 19
Suicide, DIY 204
Suicide, females exceed males in China 175
Suicide, high female rate in Sri Lanka 175
Suicide, high incidence in European Jews under Nazis 173-7
Suicide, high rates in Poland and Belorussia 175
Suicide, international comparisons 175
Suicide, rate in England 175
Suicide, successful 19
Suicide, types of (table) 20
Suicide, unassisted, in elderly people with chronic illnesses 210
Suicide, very high rates in Inuit communities 175
Sulci, of brain 28, 30
SUPPORT trial 101

Supreme Court, U.S., and artificial nutrition 73

Surgeons, and occasional errors 146

Survival, duration after nutrition withdrawn 159

Suttee, in Hinduism 119

Swiss law, legality of assisted suicide since 1920s 24

Switzerland 204

Switzerland, accompanying patients to 231

Syme, Rodney, and right-to-die activism 239

Syme, Rodney, on nursing homes as 'second prison system' 239

Syphilis 14

T

Taboo about negative comments on Alzheimer's 17

Taboo, about discussing aspects of dementia 105

Terminal cancer, and overtreatment 85

Terminal sedation 112

Terminal sedation, in France 85

Terminal, meanings of 99

Testamentary capacity 45

Thanatoriums 209

Thatcher, Margaret 50

The Silent Scream, film 143

Torquemada, Tomas de 121

Toynbee, Polly 162-3

Transport, to Switzerland, and need for special arrangements 207

Tube feeding 109

Turner, Matthew, Dr, first British atheist 122

Tutu, Desmond, Archbishop, supports MAID 117

U

U.K., opinion surveys 24

Unassisted Rational Suicide (URS) 19

Understandable misery 154

Unipolar depression 35

Urinary infection, in terminal dementia 159

V

van Gogh, Theo 15

van Gogh, Vincent 14, 15

Vascular dementia 49

Vascular dementia, blockage of arteries 30

Vascular dementia, lesions in 30

Vascular dementia, prevention of 31

Vatican, opposition to assisted dying 115

Vegan diet 35

Ventricles, of brain, enlarged 29

Visual impairments, and signing documents 207

Vitamin B12 deficiency 35

Voluntary euthanasia 11, 19, 22

Voluntary Euthanasia Society 97, 138

Voluntary Euthanasia Society, and first Guide to Self-Deliverance 213

Voluntary Euthanasia Society, and Jewish refugees 174

Voluntary euthanasia, advantages of 23

Voluntary stopping of eating and drinking (VSED) 111, 219

W

Wain, Louis 14

Warnock, Mary, Baroness 104

Weaver, J, Sorrows of a Century (book) 19fn

West-European/Old-Commonwealth nations 181

Western Europe, attitudes to assisted dying 22

White matter, in brain 30

Whitehorn, Katherine 162-5

Widdicombe, Ann, MP 119

Will, ordinary 45

Woolf, Virginia 14

World Federation of Right-to-Die Societies 253

Yuill, Kevin 134, 144

Z

Zweig, Stefan 133

pg 109-110 Paper by Cantor

* pg 187 - "pack it in" when the
dementia reaches the
institutional stage - of
or when the quality of
life has become too poor

pg 201
pg 208
pg 239, 24_